Perfect Body

By
Roe Gallo

Perfect Body

©1997, Roe Gallo

Published By:
ProMotion Publishing
3368F Governor Dr.
Suite 144
San Diego, CA 92122

(800) 231-1776

ISBN 1-57901-024-5

Printed in the United States of America

Printed on recycled paper

Perfect Body

Photography
Jack Hutcheson, San Francisco

Make-up and hair
Sherrie Long, San Francisco and Los Angeles

Editing
Catherine Ryan

For information about lectures, consultations or training send your request with a self-addressed stamped envelope to:

Roe Gallo
P. O. Box 25512
San Mateo, CA 94402-9998

To book Roe Gallo
on radio or TV shows call
(508) 432-5880
http://home.earthlink.net/~roegallo/

Special Thanks

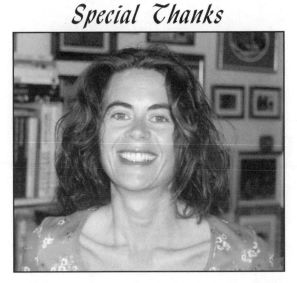

...to Catherine Ryan for her hard work doing the initial editing of the book and for her continual support and encouragement.

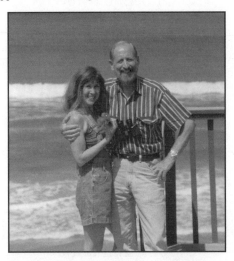

...to Ric Lambert who introduced me to my wonderful publisher. Ric has been living healthy on raw fruits and veggies since 1976. He is 68 years old and has more stamina than most 30 year olds.

Dedication

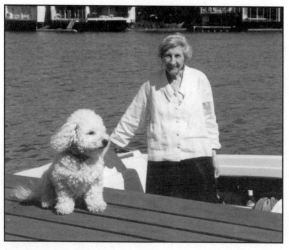

This book is dedicated to my husband, Greg;
my son, Jaime; my step-daughter, Alicia; and my mom, Carmela.
With lots of love.

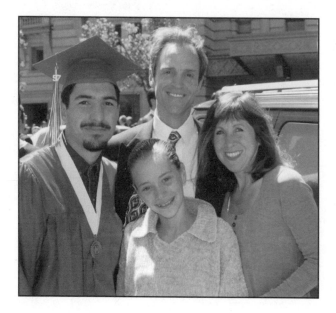

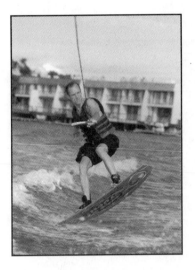

My husband Greg...

my daughter Alicia...

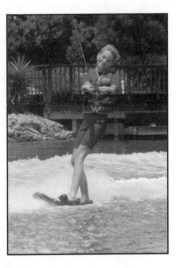

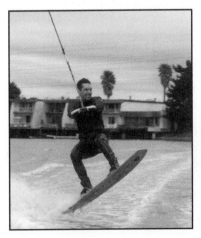

and my son Jaime are all enjoying themselves wake boarding.

Disclaimer

Roe Gallo is not a medical doctor nor does she claim to be one. She does not practice medicine because she doesn't believe in it.

Roe works with the natural functions of the body. What she says makes sense. I've seen her work with people that doctors gave up on and help them to become healthy.

Roe Gallo is my mother and for 18 years she's taught me how to take care of myself. Now you have the opportunity of having her teach you.

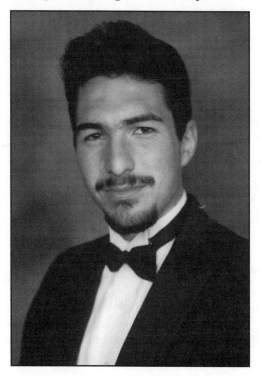

Jaime

TRUTH goes through three stages:
First, it is ridiculed;
Next, it is violently opposed; until
Finally, it becomes common knowledge.

— Discovered on a bathroom wall

Table Of Contents

Congratulations!

You've taken the first step to changing your life forever! From now on you'll never have to be unhealthy or overweight. You'll be amazed just how easy it is to be permanently lean, fit and healthy.

There are three basic reasons why most people are sick and fat — a lack of knowledge, a lack of belief and a lack of action. By the time you finish reading my book you'll have accurate information, new beliefs and a plan of action so that you can live the rest of your life lean, fit and healthy.

If you want to have a perfect body this book is for you regardless of your age or sex. You don't have to live with bad skin and excess fat, or the common diseases and conditions of aging. And, you don't have to be tired all the time. All these things that seem natural — are not. They seem natural because they're common but I'll prove to you that they are all unnatural conditions. And, I'll show you that all these symptoms are totally preventable and reversible.

When you finish this book and do the simple things I suggest, your life will be incredible! You'll have more energy to have more fun — more then you ever imagined possible.

Different from anything else, The Roe Gallo Way is *easy* and *permanent*—I guarantee it!

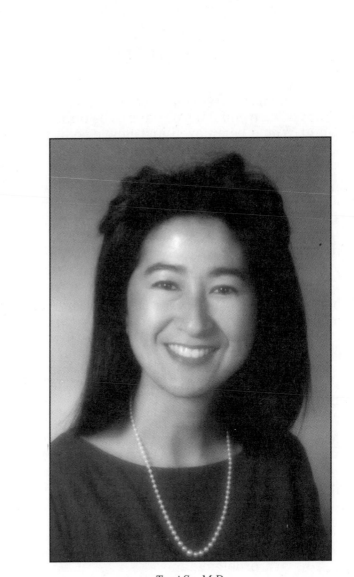

Terri Su, M.D.

Foreword

As a medical doctor I have spent years training in the various treatments of the normal and abnormal afflictions of the human body. And, as a medical doctor, I have experienced first hand the long term ineffectiveness and often damaging results of these treatments. Over the years, a frustration has grown inside me, a frustration with the symptomatic approach of modern medicine. So much attention has been paid to disease that the entirety of the solution has been missed. In my search for a better approach I met an inspiring teacher, Roe Gallo.

Roe had also experienced ineffective and dangerous treatments practiced by the medical establishement, but from a patient's point of view. She had suffered for many years as a child and young adult with chronic asthma and frequent bouts with illness. After almost losing her life to an allergic reaction and the subsequent medical treatment, she sought out a new way of achieving optimal health. Roe has compiled in her newest and best book so far, *Perfect Body*, an amazingly elegant and common sense approach to true health that begins at the cellular level. Though Roe is not a medical doctor, her understanding of human physiology is self-evident, scientifically accurate and supported by an advanced degree and meticulous research. Her ability to write and speak clearly allows us all to grasp the sheer magnificence of our physical selves as she teaches us how to take care of the human machine. She outlines in *Perfect Body* the cause and treatment of many of society's plaguing health problems and gives us inspirational case histories of those that she has inspired to achieve optimal health and full recovery from major and terminal illnesses.

In my own life and medical practice I have sought ways to achieve true health, to not just temporarily suppress symptoms with medication but to enable the body to heal itself as was intended by design. Roe shows us the way and lives it as an example. Her passion for truth radiates from the pages and immediately instills within us confidence in her message. There is no element of faddishness in this message and she doesn't offer a quick fix to our problems. She lays out on the table the facts and tells us that if we want to have energy, vitality and freedom from illness and excess weight then we must make a permanent change in our lifestyle, a holistic change that will address our physical, spiritual and mental health. This is what has drawn me to Roe. She doesn't mince words or nurture our excuses — she tells us the truth.

Within the following pages I have no doubt that you will be astounded by the simplicity of the solution Roe lays out, and probably intimidated at first by the lifestyle change that will be required. But keep in mind that the results are truly amazing and that the changes in your lifestyle will be fun, exciting and empowering. Roe's message is revolutionary and addresses not only our internal well being but the well being of the planet. Congratulate yourself for taking the first step on your journey to achieving your *Perfect Body*.

Terri Su, M.D.
Sebastopol, CA

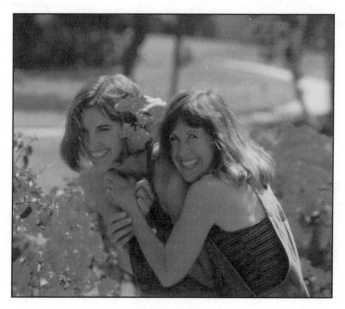

Deanna and Roe

Introduction To Roe

Throughout our entire lives, the majority of us have entrusted our health and well being to the hands of our doctors. We grow up believing that the medical profession is the *only* authority on health. I, like you, was no different until the day I met Roe Gallo. What seemed to be a normal day in graduate school turned out to be a day that was to change my life forever. Roe Gallo's powerful information not only transformed my life but it saved the lives of both of my parents. Our testimonies are included in this book.

Perfect Body is required reading for anyone committed to increasing the quality of their lives. I have personally witnessed the enormous impact this information has had on Roe's clients. I have witnessed Roe work with people who the medical community had given up on and transformed them back to perfect health. Her commitment, passion and true desire to better people's lives is apparent in everything she does. The answers to obtaining perfect health are in the pages of this book. This is truly the best and only guide for the perfect body. Roe has provided you with a step-by-step process guaranteed to show results like you would never have imagined.

I cannot properly express how much I admire Roe Gallo for her incredible work in educating the world on true health. I see Roe as a leading authority in the field of nutrition and health. It is very rare that a person comes into my life and has such a profound impact on it. I owe Roe so much. I love her like a sister and I promise you that the information you are about to read will change your life forever. Throughout my seven years in college, nothing has impacted my life like the information on the pages of this book.

Deanna Latson
San Diego, CA

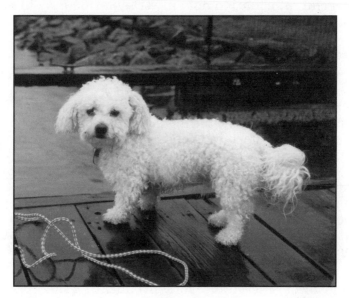

Biji

Preface

My Passion

Why do I have such a passion for this subject? Because I'm *alive* today. And I'm not just barely alive. I'm incredibly alive. I have more fun and more energy than anyone I know. I'm happy. I'm healthy. And, I have a dog. This may sound silly to you because a lot of people have dogs. But I never had one. Every time I got near a dog or a cat, my eyes would tear, I would sneeze and wheeze, my chest would hurt and my throat would itch and start to swell. But no more. Now, Biji, that's my dog's name, sleeps in my bed. And, I can play with any animal without so much as a sniffle.

All my childhood I was sick. I spent most of my younger years in bed or visiting the doctor. I suffered from severe, constant colds and several bouts of pneumonia. I couldn't live the lifestyle my friends took for granted. I couldn't run and play with the "normal" kids because my asthma was so bad my chest would constrict with pain and I would wheeze and gasp for breath. I was a chronic asthmatic. I was allergic to dust, animals, pollen—almost everything.

Doctors injected me with whatever the pharmaceutical companies were pushing that year. On days when I was well enough to go to school, I carried an inhaler and a well-stocked pill box. I was a walking medicine cabinet. I endured chronic eczema, an irritating and embarrassing condition requiring medicated soaps, special lotions and artificial light applications, among numerous other "treatments."

At six, I found a way to deal with my pain. I imagined moving the pain throughout my body and finally out through my fingertips. I practiced this continuously until the pain would actually disappear for brief periods of time. Although I didn't know it at the time, I was learning self-hypnosis and I was fairly successful! As my mastery of this process increased, I amazed my doctors and dentists. Later, as an adult, I had gum surgery and a tooth extracted *without* the aid of anesthesia or medication. With the increased ability to control my pain came a kind of freedom.

In high school, I tried out for the basketball team, but was turned down because of my asthma. At that disappointing moment I decided I would never miss another day of school because of illness. During those four years of high school, I missed only 18 days and not one because of illness — wheezing or not, I went to school.

Because of my limitations, I learned patience and developed a great appreciation for things most people take for granted. I remember spending hours trying to force my asthmatic lungs to breathe deeply, dispelling the pain. Days without sinus headaches were blessings.

My biggest lesson came when I was twenty five, a time in my life when my feelings of self-control were challenged. I had taken courses in self-hypnosis and parapsychology and had studied western psychology and mind control. My health was improving. I had practiced yoga (hatha) and was a semi-vegetarian (I still ate fish and dairy products).

One day, while eating breakfast with a friend, she offered me a taste of her buckwheat pancakes. Within minutes I had a severe allergic reaction. Terrified, I forgot all of my self-control skills; I became a helpless child again. Within thirty minutes I was in an emergency room being injected with adrenaline. After the adrenaline took effect I was given aminophylline, a new asthma drug. The next thing I remember was being slapped and yelled at; the group of doctors surrounding me had administered more adrenaline. My heart had stopped. I had reacted negatively to the aminophylline.

When confusion and self-doubt descend, fear wins out. Like others in our culture, I was conditioned to put my faith and trust in doctors rather than in myself. Having taken the trust-in-others route during my allergic reaction, I continued to follow their dictates. Several hours after arriving in the emergency room I was transported to the pulmonary ward for further treatment. At the time of my admittance I could walk, but after less than two weeks in the ward I could barely push my own wheelchair. By the end of the third week my pain was so great and my breathing so shallow I couldn't even wheel myself down the hall. I asked the doctors why I was getting worse, but they told me not to worry — that I would improve in time. I felt dismissed and intuitively knew that they were wrong. I asked about my medication. Once again I was told not to worry and they gave me no information. I was terrified, watching and feeling my body fall apart. So, I decided to investigate.

I listened to my intuition. I knew this was a question of survival. I asked a fellow patient to wheel me to the nurses' station and, when no one was looking, examined my chart. The doctors were prescribing an oral dose of aminophylline that, when injected, had caused my heart to stop. The next morning I questioned my medical team. They told me they were aware that the drug was the same but they considered it the best medication for me. They said the small, oral dose I received would not affect me as had the larger, intravenous dose. My whole being went into red alert: a slow death versus a fast one! I needed to take control in order to save myself.

Acting on my intuition and against my conditioning, I stopped taking all the medications. I visualized the pain leaving my body. I took long showers and visualized my lungs clean. I drank large quantities of water to flush the drugs from my system. I ate only the fruits and vegetables that my friends brought to me. I never told anyone at the hospital what I was doing.

With each passing day my medical team remarked on the wonderful progress I was making. I said nothing but continued my regime. Within one week I could walk well enough to sign myself out of the hospital. My doctors became upset. They couldn't understand why I wanted to leave when I was finally improving. They revoked my decision. Informing them of my legal rights to leave, I also revealed my health regimen and gave them my opinions about their methods — that their ideas were illogical and ineffective and life threatening. I was still in pain but I managed to get out of the hospital, against the advice of my doctors and against the wishes of my family.

Since my pain and physical symptoms continued, I again sought medical care. I went to see a pulmonary specialist at the University of Pennsylvania. There, in desperation, I once again gave up control of my health to the medical community. I was given a prescription for a cortisone drug and each time I took it, I initially experienced a day or two of relief. But by the third day, my pain would come back and breathing would again become difficult. To combat this, my doctor increased the dosage. I continued this treatment plan for three weeks. But I was in pain, still wheezing and I was beginning to bloat. Once more I thought it necessary to explore the therapy chosen for me. In the Physician's Desk Reference (PDR) I discovered that predisone, the cortisone drug I was taking, was classified as a" dependent" — the more I took the more my body needed for survival. Eventually, it would kill me.

I knew this meant that if I were to take charge of my life I also would be taking charge of decisions concerning my death. The next day I called my specialist to question him about my findings and to ask him if, by sticking to his plan, I would have to resign myself to a life, a short life at best, of drug use. He confirmed my suspicions but warned me that I would die without the assistance of the drug.

We ended the conversation. Suddenly I recalled a course I'd recently completed in critical thinking. I had perused many media sources to find errors in logic and had received an A in the class. Now it seemed time to apply my learning to my life.

I threw out the pills!

Contrary to all professional advice, I believed I could become healthy and I began to suspect that there was a lesson I needed to learn about the cause of my illness. I took a good look at my past. I had begun a transition to vegetarianism at twenty one. It was then that my energy level improved tremendously and many symptoms of my ill health had disappeared. Alarmed by the most recent death sentence at the hands of my pulmonary specialist, I weighed the information I had gathered and concluded that the only logical way I would heal would be through fasting — in order to quickly purge my body of its worst stored-up toxins. I acted on my conclusion.

That was the most frightening thing I have ever done. I had always listened to doctors. I grew up on medications. Now I knew more than ever that I had to take full responsibility for my life and for my death. I knew I had to go with my intuition and trust my thinking. I was compelled, by my own experiences and studies, to choose a route running against all medical advice.

Taking ultimate responsibility for my own body, for my life or death, was new to me. The first three days of my fast were hell. I actually thought I might die. I couldn't tell which was worse, the pain in my chest or the pain in my head. I drank only water — and I had to literally crawl to my kitchen to get it. On the fourth day, I experienced a little relief from the pain and could actually walk to the kitchen.

I did a two week water-only fast and after two weeks — where was the asthma? Not in my *body*. After 25 years of pain and suffering and even coming so near to death, it only took my body two weeks to clean up the asthma. I can still remember the first deep breath I took without pain. I cried.

I am alive today because I followed the three simple steps that will be presented in this book. I didn't have a choice. Don't wait until you don't have a choice.

Special Acknowledgment

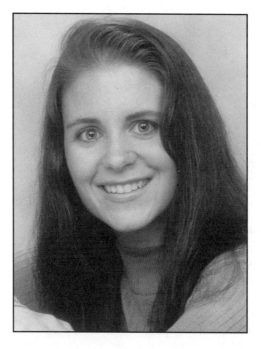

...to Kimberly Perkins for her compassion, understanding and incredible patience in taking "Perfect Body" from a typed manuscript to a completed book.

What Is A Perfect Body?

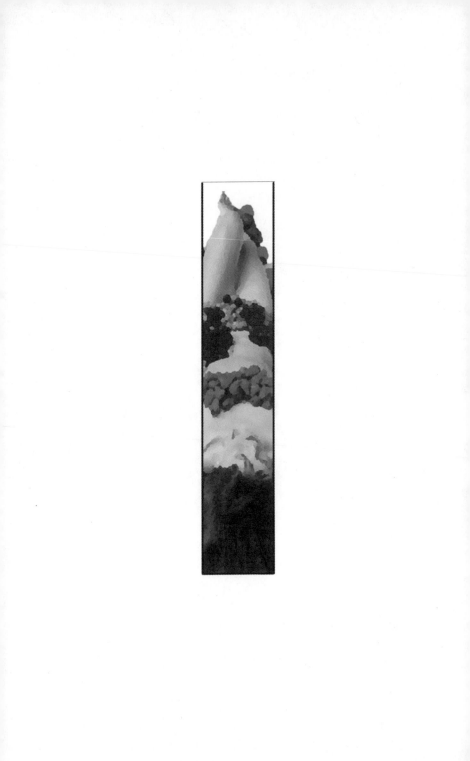

1

WHAT IS A PERFECT BODY?

What pictures come to your mind? A beautiful model on the cover of Cosmopolitan? Why? Because models always look good. They look healthy. But it's just an illusion.

Look at my picture on the cover of this book. How do I look? Peaceful? Serene? Comfortable? I was anything but peaceful, serene or comfortable. When I posed for this photo I was on a cold concrete floor with boxes propped under my left hip and shoulder and a cellular phone wedged under my head. The fruit was cold and wet, my body was freezing, my left leg was numb and I was in pain. After more than an hour in this position, Jack, my photographer got this beautiful shot. But, it's just an illusion.

If you take care of your body just on the outside you may look good for awhile, *if* you have a strong genetic background, but the illusion won't last.

A perfect body is lean, fit and healthy. Having a perfect body means that you look and feel great. Having a perfect body means having unstoppable energy. Having a perfect body means having mental as well as physical health. Having a perfect body means being free of disease and all symptoms of disease. Having a perfect body does not mean having the illusion of beauty and health — what it does mean is radiating true beauty that comes from true health. True health is never an illusion. True health is a joy. True health is about thriving, enjoying your life, having fun!

What Is Healthy?

My cousin thought her father was healthy. When he suddenly died of a heart attack, she was shocked. "But Roe, he was so healthy. He walked every day, he stopped eating so much red meat and he took his blood pressure medicine regularly."

I met with a long time high school friend. When I inquired about her dad she said, "Oh, my dad is still the same. You remember, he never gets sick. He's 68 now and still really healthy." But when I asked her why he was living with her she matter-of-factly said, "Well the doctors thought it would be better after this last bypass operation, this was his second and it left him pretty weak."

My dear friend, Deanna, thought she was healthy although she was overweight, had migraines several times a week and was addicted to pain killers. When I started working with Ed, Deanna's father, I asked his wife Sharon if she wanted to participate in Ed's new health program. She said it wasn't necessary because she was healthy and she didn't have any of Ed's symptoms and she never got sick. Two years later she was diagnosed with breast cancer.

There are many examples of people who think they are healthy. Clients tell me all the time about how healthy they are, but when I chart their health (disease) history, I find out they have one or more of the following: allergies, constipation, heart disease, atherosclerosis, headaches, high blood pressure, diabetes, heartburn, migraines, excess fat, lethargy, insomnia and nervous tension. The list is endless. If you have any of these diseases or conditions, *you are not healthy*!

Common Symptoms And Diseases

Acne	Constipation
Hemorrhoids	Pain
Excess fat	Heartburn
Heart disease	Headaches
Allergies	Lethargy
High cholesterol	Colds/Flu
High blood pressure	Diarrhea
Atherosclerosis	Arthritis
Diabetes	Insomnia
Migraines	Joint pain
Nervous tension	Stomach pain

These diseases and conditions are really all symptoms of a body that is not functioning properly — a body that is toxic. They are so common that most people consider themselves normal and healthy if they have them. Normal should equate to natural and healthy but it doesn't. In fact, normal when it relates to health, seems to mean just the opposite of natural. These symptoms are not natural and certainly not healthy. What is accepted as normal is very unhealthy.

We can't feel great, look good and have unstoppable energy if we are sick! True health requires that our entire body be in harmony — the mind, heart, liver, blood pressure and stomach — every muscle, nerve, organ, down to the smallest cell. When we are truly healthy we look and feel great, have unstoppable energy and are free of disease and all symptoms of disease. When we are truly healthy we are free to really enjoy our lives.

Do you want a perfect body? A body that is lean, fit and healthy? A body that has energy and radiant health. A body that is free from the common symptoms of disease, such as cancer, diabetes, obesity, arthritis, asthma, allergies, heart disease, high blood pressure, atherosclerosis, candida and free from the pain that accompanies these symptoms?

There are three simple steps to a perfect body. A body that is lean, fit and healthy. Follow these steps and I guarantee that you will not suffer from the common diseases of our society. Instead, you'll look and feel great. You'll have incredible energy and radiant health and you will have a lot of fun in the process.

The three steps are:

1. Get it!

2. Believe it!

3. Live it!

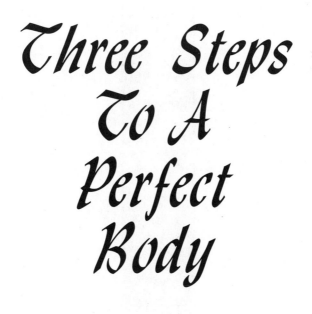

Three Steps To A Perfect Body

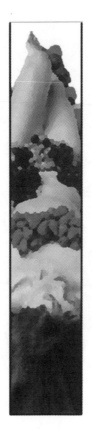

Step One
Get It

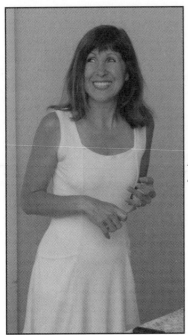

Lecturing is fun especially when friends show up.

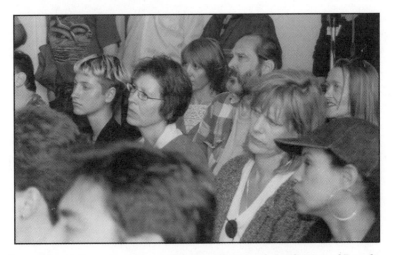

Among the audience are Simone, Maryke, Iole, David, Stephanie and Brenda.

2

STEP ONE
GET IT

Get Information

When I was 25 years old, the doctors told me I was going to die. The drugs that were temporarily keeping me from dying of asthma were already destroying me. After 25 years of trying to cure me, the doctors said I only had two choices. I could take the drugs and die a slow and painful death, or not take them and die immediately. It was not a win-win situation and I did not want to die, fast or slow but especially not slow. So I decided to look for an alternative solution. I started reading books on health. The more I read the more confused I became. Some health books totally contradicted others until all of them sounded phony. That was back in 1975 — now the health industry is even bigger and more confused. I realized that I was reading opinion and theory and not necessarily *truth*. The last thing I wanted was someone's opinion or some far out theory. I was dying. I had spent my whole life being sick. I wanted to live. I wanted to be healthy and I wanted answers.

So I studied human physiology and I got my answers. I learned about the body and how it functions. I found out about health and disease. I discovered that most disease is preventable. Degenerative genetic conditions are not preventable, but they are also rare. Common symptoms of disease such as cancer, diabetes, obesity, arthritis, asthma, allergies, heart disease, high blood pressure, atherosclerosis and candida are pervasive, preventable and totally unnecessary.

Disease And Health

The cells in your body are surrounded by fluid. This fluid is called your internal environment. Your body's main objective is to maintain balance in its internal environment because, ultimately, that's what keeps your body alive. There are many factors that affect your internal environment: the air you breathe, the light coming into your eyes, everything you put on your skin, everything you put into your mind and everything you put into your mouth. You can't always control what you breathe, what touches your skin or what you see. And you don't have complete control over what goes into your mind. But you do have *total* control over what you put into your mouth. Your health and longevity depends primarily on what you eat. What you eat determines mainly whether your body is healthy or diseased. Simple and absolute.

Everything you feed your body is broken down into nutrients and waste and transported throughout your body by way of your internal fluids. Health is maintained when you take in nutrients and eliminate waste.

When you feed your body what it needs, your internal fluids stay in balance, your cells are fed and your body is healthy. Disease, on the other hand, happens when your

14

body is overtaxed — attempting to clean non-nutritious food out of your system. Then your cells starve and eventually die and so do you. Food that does not directly benefit the body is treated as waste. It stays in your internal fluids. Some of this waste is stored in your blood as plaque and some is stored in your cells (causing some cells to either die or mutate to cancer cells). In other words, when your internal fluids are out of balance, your cells are starving, waste is not eliminated and your body is diseased. Unfortunately, this is common! Just look around and see how many people, maybe including yourself, suffer from a diseased body.

What About Fat?

I'm asked many questions about fat. Why and how do we get fat? Is getting fat part of aging? What is metabolic rate? Is there anything I can really do to prevent getting fat?

There are two basic ways of accumulating fat: by eating more than you need and by eating fatty foods.

Your body is constantly trying to do whatever it can to survive. One way it does this is by storing any excess food that it cannot immediately use. Whether it's fat, carbohydrate, or protein — it is stored as fat tissue. This way, when you cannot get enough food, your body will not starve because it can convert the fat tissue and use it as energy. By the way, you cannot reach true starvation until you first use *all* of your stored fat. Only then does your body begin to eat muscle tissue.

Does aging really have anything to do with getting fat?

Not really. When you eat too much food in general, or eat too much fat in particular, you will get fat. Age has nothing to do with it—except that the older one is, the more years one has of poor eating habits and the more one has unnaturally degenerated the body. But we can fix that.

15

Why do some people eat large amounts of food and not gain an ounce, while others, eating much less, gain weight?

This is where metabolic rate comes in. People with high metabolic rates use energy quickly, so they need more food to maintain their body functions and usually do not have enough left over to store as fat. People with low metabolic rates use energy slowly, so they need less food and they store fat immediately if they overeat. Exercise increases your metabolic rate. Usually, as people get older, they tend to exercise less. This slows down their metabolic rate. Unless their food intake decreases proportionately with their decrease in exercise, their chances of storing fat increase.

In the fitness industry, it is very common to hear trainers telling clients to do a lot of aerobic exercise so they can speed up their metabolic rate. An increase in metabolic rate allows you to eat more without gaining weight. This usually works. But it is not healthy. In the animal kingdom, of which we are very much a part, the life span of an animal is determined primarily by metabolic rate. Animals that usually live more than 100 years, such as turtles, elephants and some tropical birds, have very slow metabolic rates. Animals that usually live less than 20 years, such as cats and dogs, have faster metabolic rates. A healthy amount of exercise — enough to keep your aerobic system in good shape and your muscles toned and flexible — is good. But excessive exercise to accommodate excessive eating habits is bad.

Can you prevent getting fat?

Yes! Eat less food and don't eat fatty foods including all animal products, all cooked oils including roasted nuts, pasta sauce with oil in it, and fried foods. Eat to thrive. Get on a moderate aerobic and strength training exercise program. Then go out and enjoy how you look and feel! Your weight will take care of itself. You will look and feel *unbelievable*.

What Should You Eat?

Eat food that contains nutrients and is readily digestible. Food that goes quickly through your system gives you the energy you need and then it gets out. It's that simple. What foods are nutritious? Basic physiology shows us how and where nutrients are formed. They are created through photosynthesis.

Photosynthesis occurs in plants and trees when air, water and the minerals in the soil unite with the sun's rays to create sugar. These sugars are used by the plant for food and the excess is stored in the form of protein, carbohydrates and fats. If the plant is fruit-bearing, then these nutrients are stored primarily in the fruit. Only plants can trap and store the sun's energy and build these energy-rich and body-building compounds — carbohydrates, proteins and fats. Plants, especially their fruits, are the original source of these organic nutrients.

All of life as we know it depends upon photosynthesis. A complete supply of carbohydrates, proteins and fats are available to humans and animals through the consumption of plants, directly or indirectly. Plant eaters get their nutrients directly through plants and their fruits; flesh eaters get most of their nutrients indirectly by consuming the organ meats of plant eaters. It's crucial to realize that healthy animals, non-domesticated animals, eat their food in its raw state. Healthy animals do not consume cooked food.

Plant Eater Or Flesh Eater?

Unlike flesh eaters, plant eaters do not have a natural appetite for raw organ meats. Do you? Fruit (which includes raw nuts and seeds) and plants (which includes grasses) supply plant eaters with the perfect balance of carbohydrates, proteins, fats and water. Which is more appealing — raw liver or a luscious mango?

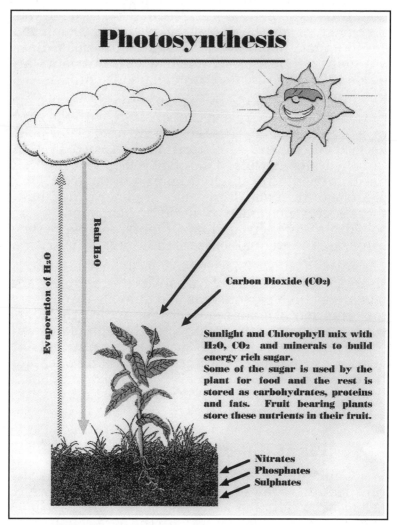

This picture is a representation of how photosynthesis works.

Besides, if we were flesh eaters, our physiology would be similar to other flesh eating animals. It isn't!

Our teeth are short and flat, designed for mashing. Our jaws move up and down and sideways. Flesh eaters, however, have long, pointed teeth for biting and ripping. Their jaws have only a hinge, allowing for an open and shut movement. Flesh eaters also have a highly acidic digestive system, allowing them to break down and assimilate highly acid-forming foodstuffs, such as meat, fish and eggs — animal foods contain the greatest amounts of acid-forming substances. Plant eaters have an alkaline system. It is extremely difficult for us to digest animal proteins even in their raw state.

If we were meant to be flesh eaters our physiology would be enhanced by the digestion of animals. But that's not the case. When we eat animals our bodies suffer. Animal products negatively affect the body's chemistry and cause imbalances in internal fluids. This change in chemistry inevitably creates disease and is compounded when the animal products are cooked. Cooking animal products dramatically alters their chemistry making them totally indigestible.

Even the scientific community has finally produced evidence that eating animal products increases the incidence of cancer, heart disease, osteoporosis and hormonal imbalances. Also, higher concentrations of chemicals and pesticides are found in livestock, more than in vegetation, because toxins are stored and build up in the systems of animals. Chemically laden foods absolutely cause neurological disorders and birth defects.

The digestion of animal products in the human body is extremely slow and incomplete, causing unnecessary and dangerous stress. The key word here is *incomplete*. Undigested foodstuffs are difficult to eliminate and so they pollute your body's internal environment.

Undigested protein causes physical toxicity. Proteins which remain in the stomach too long cause an overproduction of harmful bacteria and the undigested materials are absorbed into the blood. Depending on the metabolic rate and capacities of the individual, waste matter can accumulate in the blood vessels, eventually hardening into dangerous and toxic material called plaque. Atherosclerosis is a common cardiovascular disorder caused by the consumption of animal products.

If we were truly flesh eaters we would have a strong desire to kill animals and eat their dead bodies with our bare hands, deriving sensual pleasure from the experience as flesh eaters do — the same kind of sensual pleasure we get, instead, from eating a ripe, sweet peach, a papaya, a mango or an avocado.

Imagine yourself on a island full of beautiful fruit trees, lush grasses, animals, birds, insects, fish and other creatures. You get hungry. What would you be most inclined to eat? Would you rip into a cow, a pig, a bird, or a fish with your bare hands and eat its raw flesh or organ meats, then loll around gnawing on its bones? Would you suck on a cow's udder? Snack on some insects? Graze on the grasses? Or, would you pick a mouth-watering, sugar-sweet, luscious piece of fruit from one of the trees? The solution to all health problems is logic. Think about it!

Cholesterol

If you're confused about cholesterol, join the club. Most people are. With all the conflicting, special-interest sponsored propaganda available, there is good reason to be confused. People often ask me if eating avocados causes cholesterol build-up. *The only dietary source of cholesterol comes from animal products;* not from avocados, nuts, or even vegetables oils.

All of your cells need cholesterol. It is necessary for your survival and here are some reasons why.

Cholesterol is used to synthesize all steroid hormones. In your skin, it is used to form Vitamin D3 and, in the outer layer of the skin, cholesterol helps minimize the evaporation of body water and also helps to make your skin waterproof. Cholesterol is abundant in your nerve tissue and is instrumental in your digestive process.

Some cells manufacture their own cholesterol but the majority of your body's cholesterol is manufactured in the liver. The liver then sends the cholesterol to cells that cannot make their own by way of low-density lipoproteins (LDL's), the main cholesterol carriers. The liver also sends out high-density lipoproteins (HDL's) to remove excess cholesterol from your cells. The liver, in combination with the cholesterol receptors in the brain, creates cholesterol and then keeps it at a balanced level.

This is where special interest groups manage to make the cholesterol issue confusing. According to media reports, LDL is bad cholesterol and HDL is good. But, if your liver didn't use LDL's, your body would not get the cholesterol it needed to maintain balance. However, if you produce more cholesterol than your HDL's can remove, you're in trouble!

Genetic hypercholesterolemia is the excess production of cholesterol by the liver — it's rare. People who are diagnosed with a genetic malfunction of the liver, usually die of atherosclerosis before they reach the age of 20.

However, if your liver is functioning properly and you have no signs of genetic hypercholesterolemia, the way you get too much cholesterol is by eating animal products.

When cholesterol is ingested by eating animal products LDL-cholesterol accumulates in the arteries, the small tubes that carry blood to the heart, brain and other organs, causing them to narrow. This condition is

They're Selling Death

Did you know that the only dietary source of cholesterol is animal products?

Medical research shows that dietary cholesterol leads to atherosclerosis.

Atherosclerosis is the major cause of heart attacks and strokes.

Heart attacks and strokes are the top two killers in the United States today.

Are the poultry, meat and dairy industries selling *DEATH*?

Three times a week

They're selling *DEATH*

Meat is what's for dinner

They're selling *DEATH*

Got milk?

They're selling *DEATH*

Are you supporting industries that are *KILLING* you?

known as atherosclerosis and is the primary cause of heart attacks and strokes and also happens to be the leading cause of death in the United States today!

The good news is that you can get rid of it. Atherosclerotic plaque, which consists of cholesterol and undigested fats and proteins, begins to dissolve when animal products are eliminated. Animal products include all meats, eggs, milk, cheese, yogurt, butter, gelatin, lard — all products of animal origin. Get rid of animal products and you'll get rid of all cholesterol problems — dramatically reducing the chances of having a heart attack or a stroke.

Protein

But where do you get your protein? Do you find yourself asking this question? First of all, at what stage in your life did you need the most protein? When you were a baby and growing at a rapid speed, right? Babies get their nutrients from mother's milk. Mother's milk contains approximately two percent protein at the start of lactation. It gradually tapers down to about one percent after six months and to less than one percent after one year. Almost 90 percent of mother's milk is water, less then one percent fat and the remainder is made up of carbohydrates — simple sugars. Do young children, teenagers and adults need more protein than babies? No way. The protein myth was created in error and pushed by the meat, egg and dairy conglomerates for one simple reason:because this mythology is immensely profitable.

Are You Eating Poison?

If you eat food that is not completely digestible it *never* becomes a nutrient. Since it offers no nutrition to your body, it is processed as toxic waste. The accumulation of waste in your body pollutes it just as the accumulation of trash pollutes the earth.

23

Poison List

Poison is any substance that is not inherent, or natural, to the state of your internal environment.

Animal products

Salt

Sugar

Cooked/processed foods
This includes roasted, steamed, fried, baked, dried, stir-fried, heated, boiled, fermented, saturated fats and chemicals such as pesticides and fertilizers.

Drugs
Alcohol, nicotine, caffeine, recreational, over-the-counter and prescription drugs. These substances are not inherent or natural to the state of your internal environment — they are *poison*!

Your cells are comparable with the planet's vegetation. Polluted water supplies destroy vegetation and if this process goes unchecked, the planet's life forms will eventually die. When your body's internal environment is undernourished and polluted, your cells are destroyed until ultimately your body dies.

Poison is any substance that is not natural to your internal environment. Animal products, salt, sugar, cooked and otherwise processed foods including all roasted, steamed, fried, baked, dried, stir-fried, heated, boiled and fermented foods, saturated fats, chemicals such as pesticides and fertilizers and drugs such as alcohol, nicotine, caffeine, "recreational," over-the-counter and prescription, are not inherent, or natural, to the state of your internal environment — they are *poison!*

Your internal fluids are poisoned when you ingest these substances. And what do you think this poison in your internal environment does to your cells? *It destroys them!*

The consumption of poison perpetuates disease, eventually leading to death from disease. Being healthy, at least physiologically, means maintaining a healthy internal environment, period!

What Do I Eat?

I eat mostly fruit. Approximately 90 percent of my diet is fresh, organic fruit. I eat what's in season, so the type of fruit that I eat varies. I usually eat three pounds of fruit a day. That's approximately the weight of six apples. In the fall I eat apples, pears, avocados, dates and other seasonal fruits. In the winter I eat fresh grapefruit, navel oranges, tangerines and persimmons. In the spring, I eat valencia oranges, mangos, cherimoyas, avocados and strawberries. In the summer I have to be careful not to overeat because so many wonderful fruits are in season at the same time — grapes, peaches, nectarines, melons, figs, tomatoes, avocados, apricots — the list seems endless. I feel great eating this way and my food always tastes incredible.

This may not seem normal to you but it's as natural as it gets. And, it makes sense. Fruit provides you with the organic nutrients supplied by nature. Remember how photosynthesis works — plants trap and store the sun's energy and build the high energy and body building compounds of carbohydrates, proteins and fats for your total nutrition. Plants, especially fruit, are the original source of these organic nutrients.

I eat fruits because they provide the body with a full spectrum of nutrients and they're *so* delicious. The high water content makes fruit easy to digest — less work for the body, so you get a greater energy ratio. Even the avocado is approximately 80% water. Avocados, tomatoes, cucumbers, squash and peppers are fruits and corn is a seed.

What about nuts and seeds? With the exception of corn, nuts and seeds although botanically classified as fruit, have an extremely low water content, making them much harder to digest. Eat your food for its ease of digestibility and high nutritional and high water content.

What About Minerals?

Isn't the soil depleted? How do you know if you're getting enough minerals? If you eat fresh, organic, seasonal, fruit, it should be sweet and full bodied. If your fruit tastes great, then the mineral content is high. You can even get good tasting fruit, in spite of chemical fertilization of the soil, if the soil is not depleted of minerals. However, organic soil with high mineral content is the way to go for both great taste and nutritional benefits without toxic poisons. Again, if you look to your physiology, you find that your body needs traces of minerals to maintain proper balance, *not* mega doses. Remember, the vitamin and mineral companies are in the business of making money, not creating health. True health is much simpler. Animals in the wild are not measuring and grinding up minerals to meet any arbitrary daily requirement. They're eating what they were naturally designed to eat.

Impact On Nature

If you attempt to dominate and override nature, you are overlooking a crucial, natural law — don't mess with Mother Nature!

When you eat animals, commercial produce or processed foods, you poison yourself and the earth.

This unnatural way of living adds to deforestation, erosion, contaminated water supplies, fossil fuel consumption and the list goes on — contributing to devastating pollution.

These careless actions will probably not destroy the planet. Instead, the earth creates whatever is necessary to maintain balance. Natural disasters, such as earthquakes, hurricanes, floods, fires and electrical storms, are all part of nature's methods of restoring balance. Natural forces are oblivious to human life, achievements, possessions and lifestyles.

So instead of worrying about destroying the earth, you need to look at how you strain nature's balance and destroy yourself in the process.

Take responsibility. You can make a difference. Eat a diet that benefits you and the planet.

Eating fruit aligns you with nature. Think about it. Fruit is the offspring of the plant and it has a seed. You eat the fruit, the plant still lives and the seed goes back to the earth to either compost or grow again.

Remember you have complete control over what you put into your mouth. When you eat fresh organic fruit, you become healthy and vibrant and a living example for others.

Your example will set off a snowball effect and more and more people will buy organic thus creating a demand.

This demand will force businesses to change. Because, as you already know, businesses are in business to make a profit.

Don't just go out and join a group. Take personal action right now and be a living example.

Good-Bye Recipes

I am purposely not including any raw food recipes because we need to keep our digestive system efficient. Eating a mish-mash of food combinations, even if they *are* raw, will give you indigestion, create toxic material and gas and you will not assimilate the necessary nutrients from your food. Flatulence is not healthy!

Ideally, eat only one food at a time. Next best, combine like foods. Sweet fruits with sweet fruits, citrus fruits with citrus fruits and always eat melons alone because they just don't seem to digest well with anything else. All fruits are delicious. Once your taste buds purify, along with the rest of your body, each bite of fruit will taste incredible. You won't need to mix anything. Just wait and see! Eat your food for its nutritional content and ease of digestibility. Eat what's in season. If you are looking for variety there are many different kinds of fruits to choose from — each one a gustatory delight. Get further variety from other aspects of your life — travel, sports, dance, clothing, hobbies. Soon you'll be able to enjoy all these things much more, unhindered by the toxicity of disease.

Eat food for the energy you need in order to live your life to its fullest!

Eat to live.

Before you eat anything
Ask yourself...

- ◆ Is it fruit?
- ◆ Is it raw ?
- ◆ Is it ripe?
- ◆ Is it organic?

Perfect Food
For The Perfect Body

Organic fruit is the most perfect food for human consumption. It supplies your body with all the necessary organic nutrients and water you need to create energy. Ripe fruit is completely digestible. Organic fruit, ripe and in its natural raw state, leaves no trace of toxic waste for your body to store. Fruit keeps your internal fluids in balance. Fruit has the bacteria and enzymes necessary for your body to synthesize vitamins. Fruit contains the amino acid chains your body needs to build its perfect level of proteins. Fruit keeps your body healthy. Fruit is the perfect food for the perfect body.

Too Much Sugar?

The body needs sugar (carbohydrates) to make glucose. If you don't have enough carbohydrates in your diet, your liver will produce the glucose you need to keep your blood sugar level in balance.

When you eat carbohydrates your blood sugar level rises and your pancreas secretes insulin into your blood. The insulin signals your liver to stop producing glucose. However, if you eat concentrated sugars, your blood sugar level becomes too high, too fast causing your pancreas to produce more and more insulin and become overworked. If your pancreas cannot secrete enough insulin to keep up with your body's sugar levels, your liver does not get the signal to stop producing glucose, therefore your liver continues to produce glucose even though your blood sugar levels are already high. This puts your blood sugar levels way out of balance and your life in danger.

People with diabetes, hypoglycemia and candida are told not to eat fruit. They don't eat fruit because of its sugar content, yet they'll eat candy, bread, cake and drink alcohol. Does this make sense to you? Fruit is over 80% water and its sugars are simple and easy to digest. Candy, cake, anything with refined sugar, bread, pasta, alcohol are sometimes well over 50% concentrated sugar which is difficult, if not impossible, to digest. These substances are toxic. They absolutely damage your pancreas and take your blood sugar levels way out of balance. Also, they do damage to your immune system causing the spread of cancer and harmful bacteria. These *foods* are poison.

Eating fresh fruit — and not eating concentrated sugar or complex carbohydrates, like bread — will keep your blood sugar level in balance and your immune system working properly.

Detoxing

What if you've been on a standard American diet and your body is already a toxic waste dump? Then it's important to stop or slow down your digestive system to give your body time to clean house on a cellular level.

To cleanse the body, I usually recommend fresh squeezed, organic orange juice for clients who are not ready to do a water fast. Fresh squeezed means that you squeeze it yourself or someone does it for you *when you are ready to drink it*. I will not water fast someone unless they can commit to complete rest and I can be there to oversee the fast.

Orange juice works great because it is mostly water with a small amount of carbohydrates — simple sugars. On this program your body can start to cleanse slowly and you can still function, carrying on with work and whatever else you have going on.

Feeling Worse Before Feeling Better

The process of deep cellular housecleaning is not always totally pleasant, especially if you are very toxic. Headaches, colds, fever, skin eruptions, bowel problems, tiredness, weakness, nervousness, irritability and depression are some of the possible symptoms of toxic elimination. But hang in there. As your body begins to detoxify, the symptoms will disappear and you'll feel *incredible*.

When you stop ingesting stimulants, such as coffee, tea and chocolate, your body takes the stored caffeine and theobromine out of the cells and throws them back into the bloodstream for elimination. This chemical imbalance usually results in a headache. Also, the skin, your largest organ, helps with the elimination process and breakouts sometimes occur as toxins are pushed out through the skin. But don't worry, you'll look and feel so much better afterward that it will all have been very worth it.

Getting into a healthy dietary regime can actually make you feel worse before you start feeling better.

This process is cyclical — some days you'll feel good, some days you'll feel bad, until you finally come to the end of your cleansing and healing. It's critical to let the symptoms come and go without interference. If you take drugs to mask this cleansing process, or any kind of supplements, including vitamin supplements, you will start the toxic cycle again. If you stick with the process and remember it's just what your body has to do to get rid of its garbage, then soon you will be enjoying the benefits of vibrant health.

Vibrant Health

Vibrant health includes looking great as well as feeling great. This takes time to achieve. Just think of it this way: when I was 25 years old, I started changing my eating habits. But I had 25 years of poison to deal with. Twenty-five years of pollution can not be cleaned out overnight. Be patient. The body works miracles. It has worked miracles to keep you alive, in spite of your toxic build-up. But with a pure diet, the older you get, the *better* you will look and feel.

Conditioning Your Body

Exercise helps deliver nutrients into your body's tissues. The best exercises for the musculoskeletal system and the cardiovascular system are walking and water exercises — swimming and water running. These are natural, safe and effective. Most pools are chlorinated and such pool chemicals are absorbed into your bloodstream through your skin, so your best bet is walking or swimming in clean, pure water. Dancing, biking, skating, cross-country skiing and rowing are also great aerobic workouts and a lot of fun. When you move your body, your brain sends out signals to direct more blood to your muscles. The American College of Sports Medicine statistics show that our muscles receive about 21 percent of our blood flow when at rest; and, during strenuous exercise, that amount can increase to 88 percent.

The muscles and skeleton work together when you move. It is important to warm up the muscles gradually, increasing the blood flow to your muscles through stretching and slow, easy movements.

Condition your body gently and slowly. If you bought a new race car, would you gun it straight up to 180 mph? Of course not! You'd slowly break the engine in, allowing it to adjust to performing at high speeds. Your body is even more sophisticated. It needs to condition slowly, so that exercise is healthy rather than stressful.

Intensify your program as you build strength and stamina. The results will be safe and beneficial. You will achieve your goals and be capable of maintaining an extraordinarily high level of performance.

Posture

A strong and flexible back is very important — ask anyone who suffers from back pain. The backbone supports the entire body. Your backbone is your structural foundation, although you may not realize how important it is to take care of it until something unfortunate happens to you. Many of my clients have back problems ranging from minor discomforts to chronic pain and, with the exception of a few accidents, most of my clients' back problems are caused by poor posture.

Your muscles and skeleton cannot work properly if your alignment is off. Correct posture aids flexibility. Posture begins in your pelvis — where your entire back finds its support.

Neutral spine means that the pelvis and the neck are neither tipped forward nor backward and the shoulder and hip bones are aligned with each other. In this position, the spine is relaxed and comfortable. Practice finding your neutral spine position while walking, sitting, standing, kneeling, laying down and curled up in the fetal position. Keep your pelvis in a neutral spine position to eliminate most non-injury related back and neck problems, such as: sunken chests, raised shoulders, rounded shoulders, limps, chronic pain, herniated discs,

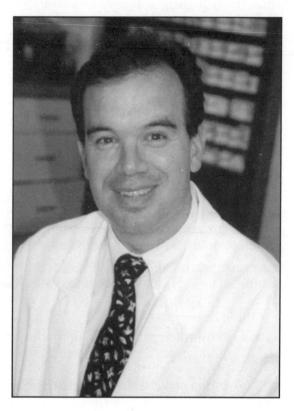

Tony

hyper-curved necks, lordosis (swaybacks), kyphosis (humpbacks) and scoliosis (laterally curved backs).

Developing an awareness of your body will help maintain a neutral spine throughout the day. Your back will gain strength, flexibility and freedom from chronic pain.

Tony

Tony was in severe pain. He could hardly walk. He went to a top orthopedic surgeon and was told that he had a herniated disc and needed surgery immediately. Fortunately, I saw Tony before he had the surgery. I explained that a herniated disc usually is caused by poor posture. I watched how he walked and held his body. Tony walked with his left foot turned out, causing his hip flexor muscles to stay contracted. The constant contraction of those muscles was pulling on the left side of his lower back and putting pressure on his disc — this pressure caused the herniated disc. Also, the herniated disc was putting pressure on a nerve, causing pain in his left leg.

Cutting out the herniated disc, which represents nothing more than a painful symptom, would not solve the problem. The cause of his pain did not start with the herniated disc. The cause of his pain started with poor posture.

His pelvis was extremely tight — he could not do a full pelvic rotation. Tony is an orthodontist and, from improperly bending over his clients, he was starting to develop kyphosis and a hyper-curved neck. Tony was 30 pounds overweight, which added more strain to his already sore back. Tony learned how to walk properly and how to sit, stand and bend. He does exercises and stretches to loosen up his pelvis and his muscles. He's lost 25 pounds and he's still losing. Tony's learning to use his body efficiently. Letting go of years of bad posture is a difficult and slow process but Tony's doing a great job.

If you are fortunate enough to have a functional spine, your primary concern should be to consciously keep it that way.

Efficient Use Of Your Body

You can build and maintain a healthy physical structure by properly using your body. Relax and look at yourself in a mirror. What do you see?

Five Posture Awareness Questions

♦ Does your pelvis tilt back (hyper-curved back, abdomen protruding and buttocks raised)?

♦ Are your shoulders rounded or raised? Is one shoulder higher?

♦ Does your chest sink in?

♦ Is your neck hyper-curved?

♦ Do one or both of your feet turn out when you walk or stand?

Thomas Hanna developed a series of exercises he called Somatics. These exercises were based on how the body, the soma, naturally works. Hanna's philosophy is that humans, although they can become victimized by physical and organic forces, can purposefully change by learning to perceive and control their internal functions. Somatic exercises reawaken the sensory motor functions in the cerebral cortex of the brain.

Sensory-motor amnesia (SMA), according to Hanna, happens when a muscle is constantly contracted sending the brain into SMA and eventually forgetting that the muscle is contracted. It takes the contracted position to be normal or "neutral." So when you go to stretch that contracted muscle the brain does not send a signal to release the muscle. This can result in a painful pull or a tear. Most importantly, the posture of the body is adversely affected. This is serious, because bad posture has long term negative effects on your entire musculoskeletal system, causing serious and, if not corrected, permanent damage to your spine, discs, joints, nerve tissue and, of course, your muscles.

Some symptoms of SMA are sunken chests, raised shoulders, rounded shoulders, limps, chronic pain, herniated discs, hyper-curved necks, lordosis, kyophosis and scoliosis. SMA can be caused by accidents, surgery and bad posture. Most alignment problems stem from poor posture. If you have any tight muscles, remember the key to successful stretching — start out with slow, easy stretches and move into holding a stretch. Always contract a tight muscle before stretching it!

Somatic exercises are practical stretches that you can incorporate into your daily routine. I highly recommend that you read Thomas Hanna's book, *Somatics*.

Three Rules For A Healthy Musculoskeletal System

- Keep your shoulders and hips even with each other and relaxed and straight.
- Keep your pelvis in the neutral position when walking, standing, siting and lying down.
- Always walk with your feet pointed straight ahead. This is important. When your feet are turned out, your hip flexor muscles are con tracted and a constant contraction of these muscles will ultimately lead to severe back problems.

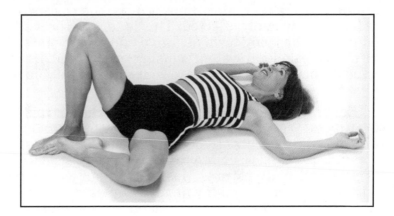

Two part pregnant lady excercise
Excellent for tight hip flexor muscles.
Go only as far as muscles will allow. Do not force knee to floor.

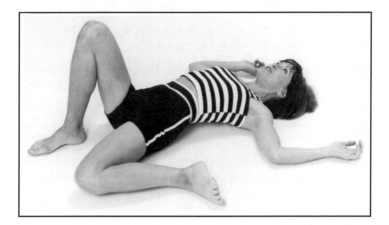

What Happens When You Exercise

Your muscles need energy to perform movement. The more you move, the more energy they need. Your muscle cells build energy molecules from the food you eat and store these molecules for future use. When your muscles move, they first use up this stored energy. If movement continues, for short durations, muscle sugar is converted to energy. When you are involved in longer term movement, more than three minutes, extra oxygen is required to make the energy you need to keep going. Oxygen fills your lungs and is then diffused into the blood. Your heart pumps this oxygen-rich blood to your muscles. If your heart is efficient, it will pump out more blood per heart beat. The more blood going to your working muscles, the more oxygen they'll have. The more oxygen, the more energy. Energy molecules are responsible for maintaining muscle contraction.

Muscles tire when they can no longer maintain a contraction. Your larger muscles will last longer than the smaller ones. So, work large muscle groups first. For example, in weight training you'd start with the back muscles, go on to the chest, shoulders and arms. In aerobic dance, the legs are worked before the arms. The intensity and duration of muscular contraction also plays a part in muscle fatigue. With regular weight training it's possible to do many more contractions than with power lifting, when the intensity is much greater and the duration of a single contraction is much longer.

There are also psychological reasons for muscle fatigue, or psychological fatigue. Psychological fatigue occurs when the brain fails to send appropriate signals to the motor nerves and the muscles fail to contract. This happens when you think you are tired. This fatigue will cause you to stop exercising even when your muscles aren't really tired.

Muscle size, strength and tendency to fatigue can be improved through both physiological and psychological exercise. Our muscles can grow in size and strength, developing specialized skills. It's important to be careful though, because misuse or overuse can physiologically stress your muscles — even causing permanent damage. Muscle training should be slow and exact. Long-duration, low-intensity exercise increases muscular endurance. Short-duration, high-intensity exercise increases the size of the muscle, thereby producing stronger contractions and increased muscular strength. This increased physiological strength must go hand in hand with psychological determination to produce maximum performance.

Four Conditions
For Healthy Exercises

- ◆ Form
- ◆ Isolation
- ◆ Tempo
- ◆ Breathing

Form

When you work your muscles you must pay attention to proper form, the isolation of specific muscle groups, the speed or tempo of your efforts and your breathing. Your awareness and care enable you to receive maximum benefits during exercise and minimize the risk of injury.

Proper form means that the exercise is done with attention to how you hold and move your body, especially the lower back, neck and joints. This is essential to the prevention of unnecessary stress in these areas. In general, the upper back and neck should be relaxed and in alignment, the lower back should be relaxed and supported and the joints should be relaxed and not locked or forced beyond a 90 degree angle. These guidelines apply during most exercises, especially when using weights. I tell my clients they may increase weights and repetitions only if they stay in proper form.

Isolation

When you isolate muscles, you focus on exercising single muscles or muscle groups, while the remainder of your muscles remain as relaxed as possible. Muscles work in pairs — as antagonists. For example, when your biceps contracts, its antagonistic or opposing muscle, the triceps, stretches. If you know which muscles perform certain actions, you can learn to isolate them.

Muscles attach to rope-like tendons. These tendons attach to bones. When you contract a muscle, its fibers pull the tendons, which in turn pull the attached bone. Picture the biceps again. When you contract your biceps, it pulls a "rope" which attaches to the radius bone in your forearm — the biceps contraction raises your forearm. On the other hand, if you contract your triceps, the biceps lengthens and your forearm extends.

Bicep curls require careful execution, especially when using weights. Your forearm and wrist should be as relaxed as possible and your shoulder held still. This helps isolate the targeted muscle. If you involve other muscles, you aren't using the targeted muscle to its maximum potential. Here's another example: during abdominal crunches, if you hook your feet to help pull yourself into the crunch, you will be using your leg muscles rather than isolating your abs. However, if you do abdominal crunches in proper form — with your head and back forming a straight line, knees bent, feet on the ground and contract only the abs to raise the body — then you properly isolate the abs. The attention to concentration on the appropriate muscles helps you reach your desired goals and decreases the likelihood of misuse and injury.

Tempo

Tempo is the rate of speed at which you exercise. If you move fast because you want to get it over with, or use momentum to help you lift or push greater weights, excess energy is used with minimum results. At a slow tempo, your muscles have to work harder — better increasing muscular strength, size and shape, as well as overall tone.

Breathing

If you pay attention to how you breathe, your blood can be fully oxygenated and your workout will be more effective. The cardinal rule is: *Never hold your breath!* Breathe out on exertion, during your working muscle's contraction; breathe in when your muscle relaxes, as it readies itself for the next contraction.

Five Steps To A Great Workout

- ◆Warm-up
- ◆Aerobic Conditioning
- ◆Stretching
- ◆Isotonics and Isometrics
- ◆Cool Down

Warm-Up With Easy Movements

Warm-up to slowly increase your heart rate so more blood can get into your muscles. The additional blood actually makes the muscles warmer, more flexible and gives them a steady increase in oxygen.

Examples of warm up activities: jog in place, slow biking, easy movement exercises.

Aerobic Conditioning

Aerobic conditioning is designed to get your heart rate up and keep it up while you are exercising. This kind of exercise needs a steady supply of oxygen-rich blood to keep going.

Examples of aerobic conditioning: biking, swimming, rowing, skating, jogging, dancing.

Stretching

Are you aware of your body enough to recognize when your muscles need to move? When babies or animals — especially cats — wake up, the first thing they do is start to move their bodies very slowly. They wiggle and squirm, they yawn and make faces and then they stretch. They're great to watch and magnificent teachers. I once heard a yoga instructor say that the best yoga teachers were cats.

When you awake, your body needs that same kind of gentle attention. Five minutes of movement and stretching can get the blood circulating and the muscles ready to start the day. Start out with slow, easy stretches, then move into holding a stretch. Always contract a tight muscle before stretching it!

Stretching lengthens your muscles and makes them more flexible. Keep your body flexible throughout busy days by periodically moving and stretching your muscles. This keeps the stresses of the day from accumulating in your neck and back and your hamstrings and lower backs won't suffer from sitting. Imagine you're a cat. Stretch every muscle of your body continually throughout the day.

Two Important Stretching Exercises

Dynamic Stretching

Start out with dynamic stretches — slow, easy, continuous movement stretches. These stretches slowly ease the muscles into a lengthening position.

Static Stretching

Static stretches are stretches that are held. Here the muscle is stretched then held in a lengthened position.

Three Excellent Stretches
For Your Back

- ♦ Knees to chest
- ♦ Cat
- ♦ Bow

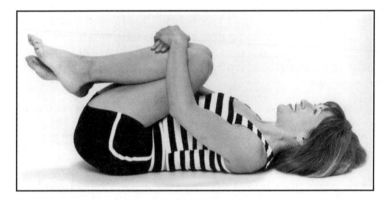

Knees to Chest

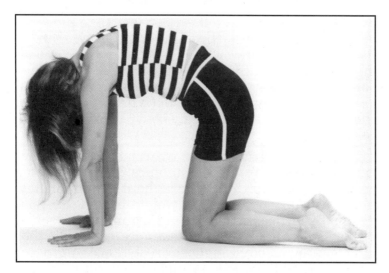

Cat stretch

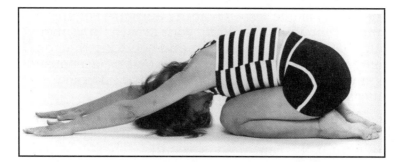

Bow stretch

Isotonics and Isometrics

My exercise routine does not just take place in a gym. I incorporate it throughout my day. Can you picture ways to work on your back and other muscles while stuck in a traffic jam? My schedule doesn't leave room for much gym time. Besides, incorporating exercises into my everyday activities makes a big difference in how I relate to my body. This is what I call the "Body Gym."

Isotonic and isometric exercises allow you to exercise almost anywhere. Isotonics can be defined as the use of equal resistance throughout a range of movement. Push-ups, pull-ups and weight bearing exercises (free or fixed resistance) are all examples of isotonic exercise. I highly recommend isotonics, especially those using your own body weight for resistance. A program of push-ups, pull-ups, squats, lunges, calf raises, abdominal crunches and pelvic tilts — all done without weights — can be incorporated in your lifestyle. No gym required. Your body is a body gym! Also, isotonic exercises can be used to strengthen the face and eyes. Facial exercise will increase your muscle tone and improve your appearance. Contracting and relaxing your eyes, strengthens your eye muscles and improves your vision. Try it. You'll be amazed.

Isometric exercises are done without movement. The key to isometrics is holding and intensifying your contraction without holding your breath. In isometrics you actually trick your brain into believing that you're doing work. In fact, whether you're pulling on or pushing against a mobile object or something stationary, your muscles work just as hard.

Isotonics and isometrics are great, especially for us baby-boomers who look for minimal investment with maximum, instantaneous results. These exercises require no financial investment and no additional time investment. The movements used are those which would

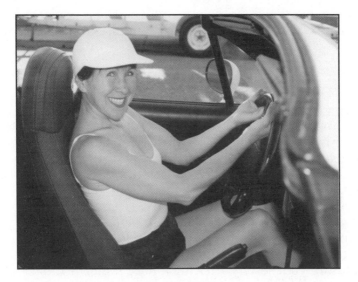

THE BODY GYM

The body gym goes where your go. These are isometric exercises using the
steering wheel for resistance.

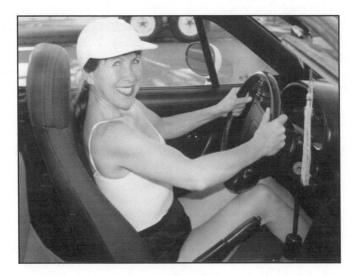

have otherwise been wasted! Isotonics and isometric are solid tools which help you achieve fitness goals gaining muscular strength, endurance and flexibility.

Stress Reduction

Using isometric exercises is another great way to relieve stress. If you are on a freeway in bumper to bumper traffic, you can stress out or you can work on your biceps, your chest, your abs. You don't need weights — use your steering wheel for resistance. You know you will eventually get to your destination. Getting stressed out won't get you there any faster, but isotonics will help strengthen and tone your body. If you focus on something other than the traffic, time will pass quickly and you'll end up at your destination feeling more relaxed and *fit*. Developing this habit takes some persistence. Remind yourself by sticking a post-it on the dash — the habit will kick in sooner than you expect!

Cool-Down

The cool-down will gradually slow down the pumping action of your heart. Remember, during exercise additional blood is being pumped to your muscles. You want this excess blood to be returned to your heart — gradually. If you stop exercising abruptly blood may pool in your veins causing pain and cramping.

Examples of cool-down activities:

Walking and stretching after heavy aerobic exercise (biking, running, etc.) and stretching after resistance exercises.

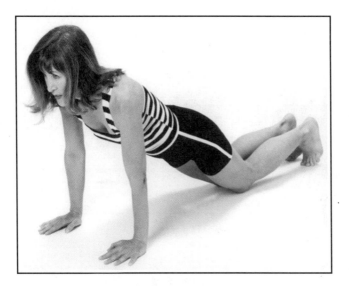

PUSH UPS
Full push-ups or with bent knees.
Neck, back and buttocks in a straight line.
Do in proper form until fatigued.

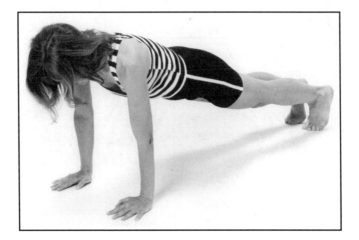

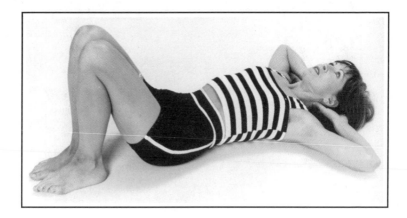

CRUNCHES
Eyes focused toward ceiling.
Neck and back in straight line.
Head rests in hands — do not pull head.
Movement comes from upper abdominal contractions.

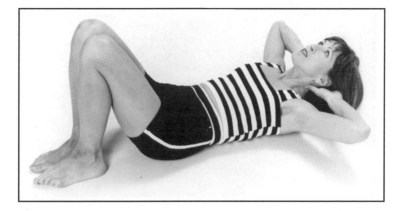

PELVIC TILT

Practice the pelvic tilt as much as possible. It can be done sitting, standing or lying down, with the buttocks on the floor or in a bridge position. The pelvic tilt is the best exercise for tightening the lower abs, toning the buttocks and strengthening the lower back.

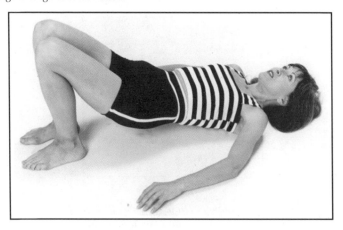

POSITION ONE
Relax on back with knees bent and feet drawn near the buttocks.

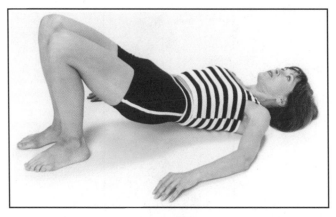

POSITION TWO
Tilt the pelvis forward by flattening the lower back. Contract the lower abdominal muscles and the buttocks. Relax back into position one and repeat until fatigued.

51

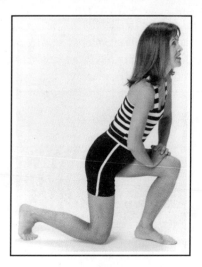

LUNGES
Place hands on waist to balance. These can be held as a stretch or done in a series until fatigued. Alternate each side. One count includes both the right and left leg.

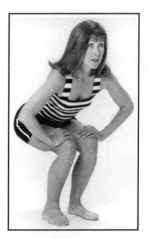

SQUATS
Do not go beyond a 90 degree bend in the knees.

Maintain the four conditions (proper form, isolation, tempo and breathing) and do the five great workout steps (warm-up, aerobic conditioning, stretching, isotonics and cool-down) and you can have a fit and beautiful body. Building a great body with your own body gym offers you the freedom to strengthen and sculpt your body regardless of where you are and affords you the safe, self-limiting resistance of your own body weight.

Correcting Your Vision

The eye muscles take much of the responsibility for good vision. If the eye muscles are tight, we cannot see distances well, leaving us near-sighted. If the eye muscles are overly relaxed, we won't be able to see well up close, leaving us far-sighted. Vision therapy relaxes and strengthens the eye muscles. Corrective glasses and contact lenses are a crutch. They help you see better temporarily, but do not correct your vision. Vision therapy *does* work, even if someone is considered legally blind. Aldous Huxley and Meir Schnieder are perfect examples. These two high-profile men went from being legally blind to being able to see by practicing vision therapy.

I wore contacts because of myopia (near-sightedness) and for severe astigmatism (irregularity of the surface of the eye). I could see well close-up, but three feet or further away from my nose, everything blurred. I also had terrible night vision. I read Aldous Huxley's book, *The Art of Seeing*, and I threw out my contacts. I started sunning my eyes. Sunning is done through lightly closed eyelids. Tilt your head toward the sun and rotate it, left and right. This allows the sunlight to gently bathe the retina. I also do palming. To palm, cup your hands over your closed eyes and visualize black. Blinking is a big part of my daily eye routine. I have a tendency to stare (the myopic stare) which causes the muscles of my eyes to stay contracted, hence the nearsightedness.

Instead of using my contact lens as a crutch, I started using my eye muscles. The first few months were challenging. I got a pair of regular glasses and wore them when I was driving, or if I otherwise really *had* to see something. My vision gradually started to improve. I read Dr. Bates' book, *"The Bates Method for Better Eyesight Without Glasses,"* as well as Meir Schneider's personal story. Schneider, who has a clinic in San Francisco, has kept his legal blindness certificate and likes to display it side-by-side with his driver's license.

I can now see the leaves on trees from a distance without corrective lenses. In the sunlight my vision is 20/20. At night I lose some clarity, especially if my eyes are tired.

I highly recommend Tom Quackenbush's new book, *Relearning to See.* Tom's book is the most comprehensive book ever written on the Bates method. If you want a simple and practical self-help book on improving your eyesight, this is the book to buy.

When I talk to clients about sunning their eyes and not wearing sunglasses they often protest. Sunglasses are particularly bad for you. The body is partially protected from the rays of the sun because of your body's natural perception of the sun's brightness. When it is sunny, the pupil of the eyes will contract, so the light is let in through a smaller opening. In the back of the pupil are melanin cells. When the sun's rays contact the pupils, the brain sends a signal to the melanin cells to release dark pigment throughout the entire body to protect the skin from sun damage. When you wear sunglasses, the darkness of the glass fools your eyes, interfering with your natural skin protection. Burning and skin cancer are the result. Use sunglasses only in dangerously intensive glare situations, such as snow skiing or driving your car toward the sun.

Surface Care

This is easy. Water is the primary ingredient. When your body is clean on the inside you need very little of anything else to keep the outside clean and beautiful.

Clean your skin with pure water. If you have a lot of chlorine in your water get a filter that gets rid of it. Bathe your skin in fresh air and sunshine. Stay away from soaps, lotions, astringents and other skin care products. If you get something on your skin that won't come off with water, like bike grease, use some fresh lemon juice or a natural cleanser on the area.

Good skin comes from the inside out. If you live in or around a big city and your skin is exposed to a lot of pollution, a little outside care might be helpful. If that's the case, rub a little avocado, cucumber, mango, papaya into your skin and notice an immediate difference. Pure cocoa butter is also wonderful.

Clean your hair with warm water and a cool rinse. Use a natural shampoo on your hair when needed. Brushing is great for your hair, it distributes natural oils, but over shampooing drys it out.

Clean your nails with warm water and a nail brush. Brushing stimulates nail growth and softens your cuticles so you can push them back. Never cut your cuticles. Don't use polish, instead buff your nails to their natural shine.

Brush your teeth and tongue at least twice a day and especially before you go to bed. I use warm water and sometimes a natural toothpaste. Floss your teeth before you go to bed. A good diet and good oral hygiene are the keys to a beautiful smile.

Smile often.

Craniosacral Therapy

Your craniosacral system consists of the membranes and fluid that protect your brain and spinal cord. It extends from the bones of your skull, face and mouth — which make up your cranium — down to your sacrum (tailbone).

The movement of your craniosacral fluid produces its own rhythm, or pulse. This pulse can be felt and evaluated to determine if your craniosacral system is in balance.

A Craniosacral Therapist uses a light touch, no more than five grams of force, to evaluate if your system is functioning properly and to influence the natural movement of the fluid to get it back into balance.

Imbalances in this system could cause sensory, motor, or neurological problems. I personally have used Craniosacral Therapy to help rid my clients of chronic back pain, migraines, temporomandibular joint (TMJ) problems and all types of physical and emotional stress. It really works.

The origin of Craniosacral Therapy goes back to the early 1900's, when Dr. William Sutherland was struck by the unusual idea that the bones of the skull were structured to allow for movement. For more than 20 years he explored this concept, eventually developing a system of treatment known as Cranial Osteopathy.

In 1970, osteopathic physician John E. Upledger observed the rhythmic movement of the craniosacral system during surgery. From 1975 to 1983, he served as clinical researcher and Professor of Biomechanics at Michigan State University. There he supervised a team of anatomists, physiologists, biophysicists and bioengineers to test and document the influence of therapy on the craniosacral system. Dr. Upledger developed Craniosacral Therapy.

I use Craniosacral Therapy on all of my clients. I find that it really helps them and they love it. They tell me it's more relaxing than a full body massage.

Train To Win

Do top athletes go to competitions unprepared? Absolutely not! Athletes train to win. Winners are prepared — physically, mentally and emotionally. They are trained to meet challenges. They know that practice and preparation are the keys to success. Beyond physical training, athletes also prepare themselves emotionally and psychologically through visualization exercises and positive self-talk. Self-talk is that little voice inside your head that says, "you can do it," or "this is too hard." You choose. Winning athletes develop the will to win and learn to anticipate victory.

Take Responsibility

If you want to be healthy, *you* have to take the responsibility for getting there. Remember, it's your life that's at risk. Make a commitment to live the rest of your life to it's fullest.

Read through my research sources listed in the bibliography if you want to satisfy a scientific mind, or do your own research. Read all the information you want, but before you make a decision regarding your life and death, look at how your body actually works. Always look to physiology. When you understand physiology, you'll understand how the most complicated medical "science" is, at times, based on fallacies.

Take responsibility *now* for your body. Apply critical thought and get accurate information. Look at all the information and most importantly, use logic before you make critical decisions regarding your life and death. Most of all — keep everything simple. It is simple.

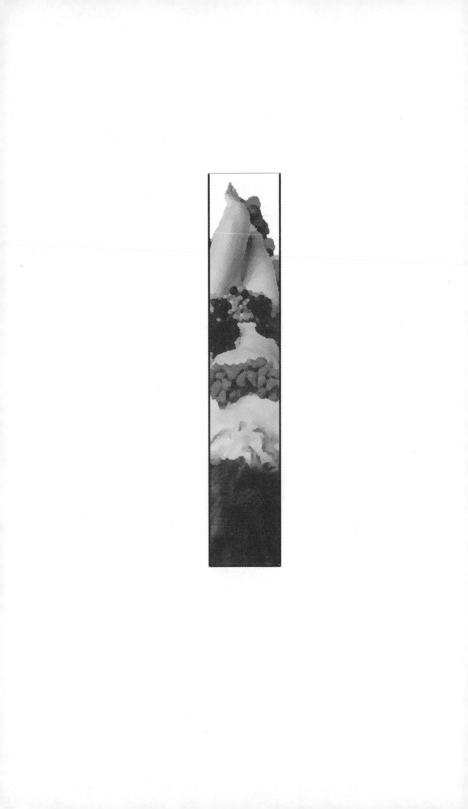

Step Two
Believe It

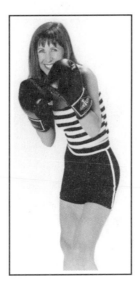

At 47, Roe is acquiring new skills. The older you get the better you get and the more fun you'll have.

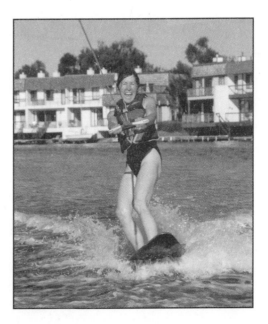

3

STEP TWO
BELIEVE IT

The Power Of Beliefs

Is there a common trait that successful people have?

Well, it certainly isn't family background. People come up from the depths of poverty and have become successful and people from wealthy families have become losers.

It's not just a matter of education, either. People who didn't finish grade school sometimes become multi-millionaires and street people sometimes hold Ph.D's.

What is it then? What separates winners from losers?

It seems there is a common ingredient in success stories and if it is missing, failure results.

This ingredient is positive beliefs.

Thoughts that come into your mind can be positive or negative and when you believe them they become things. Things that can affect your life.

Your beliefs affect your idea of who you are. This includes how you see yourself, how you feel about yourself and the value you place on yourself and what you do.

Think about this: If you don't see yourself as successful, then you don't feel good about who you are and what you are doing. If you don't place a high value on your time and your work, then you won't be successful. On the other hand, if you see yourself as successful, feel great about who you are and place a high value on your time and work then you will move in the direction of success.

Where Do Mistaken Beliefs Come From?

I had always listened to doctors. I grew up on medications. I believed in doctors and medicine. I didn't know any other way. Stepping out of old comfortable beliefs, going against the beliefs of family, friends, society, normal health education and the medical industry is scary, to say the least. You must separate yourself from the comfortable, familiar and, I must add, failing beliefs that you thought were right, so that you will have room for new beliefs that are based on a higher set of standards.

I made changes that totally went against my belief system. The research I did wouldn't have done me any good if I didn't believe it. It made sense, but if I hadn't believed it, it would have been useless.

It was a little easier for me to change my beliefs because I didn't have a choice. I would have died. But it was still scary. Most of my clients don't have a choice either. Usually people come to me after the doctors give up on them. But some of them come without symptoms and therefore without a sense of urgency. With these clients, we spend most of the sessions working on changing their beliefs.

Much of your beliefs about health and disease are formed by the food and drug industries and the billions of dollars they spend in marketing and advertising.

Also, doctors have a big impact on your beliefs. I am a great example of that. If I had continued to blindly place my faith in the medical profession, I wouldn't be here today writing this book. Most doctors are doing the best they can with information they have and many of them are truly caring individuals. But doctors don't study health, they study disease. They are taught that interference with nature, by using chemical treatments and surgery to remove or repress *symptoms*, is the way to achieve health. Again, really think about this. Does this make sense to you? Do you want to believe this backwards system? Many people do. It allows them to continue their unhealthy lives and leave the responsibility to the men and women in white coats.

Don't look to the medical industry to provide information on health because it doesn't know how to create health. All that doctors know is how to treat symptoms. The health industry, like the food and drug industries, is a *massive* money-making machine. The health industry is *excellent* at business and *terrible* at health. You need to replace harmful, erroneous beliefs with positive, productive, empowering and healthy beliefs to be healthy.

Look To Other's Success When Deciding What To Believe

My clients have rid themselves of heart disease, high blood pressure, breast cancer, throat cancer, neurological trauma, arthritis, acne, allergies, migraines, high cholesterol, ulcers—the list goes on and on and on. Of course it does. Because there is only *one* solution to *all* the symptoms of a toxic body. Detoxify!

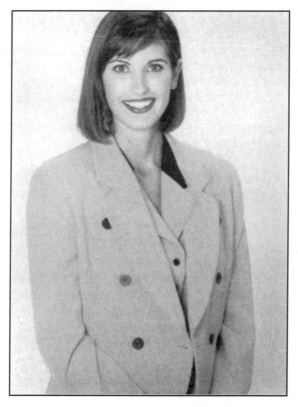

Deanna

Deanna

Deanna was 23 years old and in graduate school at San Francisco State University when I met her. She didn't feel unhealthy. In fact, she considered herself to be vibrant, energetic, enthusiastic and in great health. But she didn't know what she was missing. Now, she's reaching her real potential — which is off the chart. When we met, Deanna thought I was a fun-loving, high-energy woman, with a crazy diet. She wouldn't read my first book and was very resistant to change. Then, one night we went out and, after several hours of dancing, Deanna was exhausted while I was still going strong. She decided to make some changes.

I explained that the first step for her was to define *healthy* for herself. For the first time, she looked to what her body was telling her. She suffered from the most painful headaches anyone could imagine. She made regular visits to the doctor for prescription pain and sleep medicines. She bought so much Tylenol and Excedrin she should have purchased stock in the company. She got to the point where four pills wouldn't curb the pain, so she began taking six at a time. She was taking Vicodin to sleep at night. For those not familiar with Vicodin, it's a narcotic. It is habit forming and can have severe side effects, including the possibility of slipping into a coma. She also took birth control pills daily. After stepping back and looking at her pill intake she realized she was far from healthy and she definitely needed to redefine health for herself.

I told her that she could rid herself of the headaches and feel more energy and zest than ever before. She was a total skeptic. She says that even as a child if her dad said, "Don't sit in that chair; the leg is broken;" she would have to try it for herself and tip over. She had a hard time taking in new information and believing it wholeheartedly — this health information was no different. Although she still was not sold on the fact that she was completely unhealthy at 23, she was convinced and deeply concerned that her father was unhealthy. So, mostly for his sake, she continued her quest for information.

Starting to realize how much more to life there was, she decided to begin changing her habits and lifestyle. She attributed much of her strength to the fact that she wanted her father to consider all this new information. She didn't want to be a hypocrite. Step by step, she began eliminating unhealthy foods from her daily routine.

First on the chopping block came fast food. Next up were all meats including chicken, beef, fish, turkey, pig and every other type of animal flesh. After taking these steps, she was ready to get off caffeine. She had been drinking three double mochas a day, so this was not easy.

Her body was getting a complete and total overhaul and, as she put it, "Its only way of saying 'thank you' was by breaking out in pimples and rashes." The toxins were pouring out everywhere. She had always had clear skin until this point in her life. I explained to her that the rashes and pimples would go away after her body released the bad toxins that were causing the break-outs. Which they did.

She did not like the, "It only gets worse before it gets better" idea. But, she perservered, especially with her dad's poor health still lingering in her mind. She stopped taking medicines, including birth control pills. She stopped eating *all* animal products. She was committed to a diet of raw fruits and vegetables. The third month into this new lifestyle, she began counting the benefits. She had gone 33 days without a headache. This was truly amazing, considering that she previously suffered from headaches daily.

It has been three years and she still hasn't put a pill into her body. She no longer suffers from headaches. And, she is 40 pounds lighter. She is healthier and has more energy than she ever dreamed possible. Deanna looks truly *beautiful* and feels great and she knows she could never go back to eating the way she used to.

Ed (Deanna's Father)

When I met Ed he was 51 and "tired all the time." I'll never forget the scene in his kitchen. Deanna wanted me to work with him. She felt the urgency of his very poor health. Ed owned a horse ranch and he was always a "meat and potatoes" man. He listened very carefully as I made my proposal. Then he replied, "Forget it, there's no way that I'm going to eat rabbit food."

At that point Deanna turned to him and started to cry. She said, "If you die before your grandchildren are born, I'll *never* forgive you." He agreed to work with me for a month.

Ed had been on high blood pressure medication (Vasotec) for nearly 12 years and, even with the prescribed medications, his blood pressure was 150/90 and sometimes higher. He had also been on antacids (including Pepcid) for more than 20 years because he had acute acid reflux. His condition was so bad that he had to sleep with pillows to prop him up so that the acid did not rise into his throat. He also had a precancerous condition in his esophagus because of all the excess caustic acid. He suffered from headaches — usually migraines — on a regular basis, for which he took Vicodin as his daughter had. He was usually anxious, so he took Paxil (an antidepressant) daily.

This poor man was a heart attack waiting to happen and, for the most part, a total toxic waste dump. At 6'3" and 259 pounds, he was 80 pounds overweight, his cholesterol was extremely high (over 200) and he was usually very agitated. His diet was standard American fare, more than 90 percent cooked food, a lot of animal products, salt, sugar, cooked oils and so on.

The first thing I did was outline a diet consisting of more than 90 percent raw, organic food: fresh fruits,green leafy salads, fresh vegetables, some raw nuts and seeds. Within six months he was eating more than 90 percent fruit.

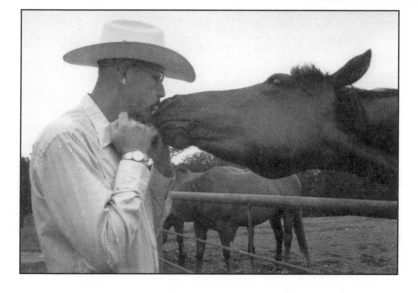

Ed

**Ten Reasons Why I Love
The Roe Gallo Diet...
AKA
The Rosemaria, Your Friends
Think Your Nuts Diet...
AKA
The Lifelong, How I hate
What I Eat Diet...**

I love this diet because:

10. My bowels work so well that I pack a porta-potty with me wherever I go.

9. My friends who knew me before the diet were already convinced I was a little off. Those same friends are now attempting to have me committed.

8. I have eaten so many bananas, I now have to climb a tree to go to the bathroom.

7. Health nut hippies are beginning to hang around my home.

6. I now have more gas than PG&E.

5. When my friends invite me to dinner I have to sit outside with the dog until they are finished eating.

4. I have pimples in places I didn't even know I had places.

3. I now choose to eat the bag the groceries came in, rather than the groceries.

2. I have consumed an endless variety of lettuce all of which tastes exactly the same.

1. Because of all the weight I have lost, it will cost me $4,866.00 to replace the clothes I can no longer wear.

He also bought a blood pressure cuff and took his blood pressure every morning before he got out of bed and every evening.

In a month, he'd lost 20 pounds, his blood pressure started to drop, he had very little acid reflux and fewer headaches.

At the beginning of the second month, he started weaning off his medications. This was a slow process, because going "cold turkey" could have put him in physical danger. The body does become addicted and dependent on such chemicals. He was taking two blood pressure medications, the acid reflux drug twice a day, the Paxil daily and Vicodin at least 5-6 times a week. He reduced his intake of the blood pressure pills and the antacids to once a day for a week then every other day for the second week and every third day for the third week. During this time I was constantly monitoring his blood pressure and it was steadily droping. Also, the acid reflux problems were gone, along with the headaches. After four weeks of the weaning process, he stopped the medication completely, except for the Paxil. His blood pressure was 110/70 with no medications.

This was just the beginning. After three months he was totally off the Paxil and after six months his weight was 179 pounds. He'd lost 80 pounds, his blood pressure averaged 115/54, he had more energy than he had in his twenties and he was calm. He still is.

No more anxiety, no more headaches. I asked him to go to his family doctor for a complete physical and his doctor was shocked. He said that he "never saw such dramatic change resulting from diet." He also told Ed to "keep doing" whatever he was doing. His doctor said he was in "better than excellent health," his blood pressure and cholestrol were low. He had the "prostate of a 20-year-old."

Ed's body just needed the opportunity to get rid of the poisons (bad food, medications, alcohol, etc.) and get on to a clean and natural program. Ed says that now he has "freedom from illness and pills for the remainder of my life — the life that I never expected to have."

Sharon (Ed's Wife, Deanna's Mother)

I met Sharon when I met Ed almost three years ago. I asked her if she was going to join Ed on his road to health. She told me that she was already healthy — she *never* got sick. She said it wasn't necessary for her to change her diet because she was doing just fine. Sharon never had any major illnesses other than a bout with hepatitis as a child. She was never hospitalized other than to give birth to her two children. Her diet consisted of just about anything she wanted and she didn't see any negative affects from her eating habits because she usually felt fine. She was about 35 pounds overweight but she felt it was normal. Weight gain was something that happens with age. Right? After all, most people her age, 52, looked and felt worse then she did.

In 1993, two years before her menopause began, Sharon's family doctor put her on estrogen. Why? She didn't know. He just told her it would be a good idea. So she followed his advice. The estrogen made her feel terrible and anxious. So, after two years, she stopped. Soon after she stopped the estrogen, she started menopause. She experienced frequent hot flashes — six to ten times a day — and heavy night sweats. These night sweats were so bad she had to get up to change her soaked sheets. Mood swings tormented her daily and she usually felt anxious. In addition to the menopause symptoms, she developed pains in both of her shoulders. The doctors weren't sure the pain was arthritis or bursitis.

Perfect Body

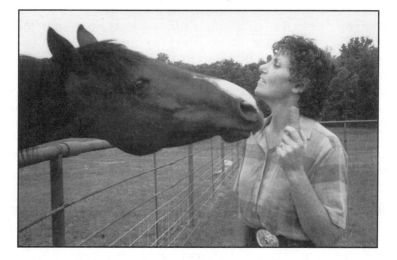

Sharon

Sharon couldn't reach above her head without hurting and her grip strength was weak, at best.

Sharon resigned herself to the fact that all women eventually had to go through menopause and have these problems. They're normal. Most of her friends had more aches and pains than she did, so she felt relatively lucky and assumed her shoulder problems were normal, too. Sharon believed, as most women do, that aches, pains and menopause symptoms were part of the normal aging process and there wasn't anything she could do about it — except take drugs to ease the discomfort.

For her shoulder pain she took several types of over-the-counter medications. The drugs gave her minimal temporary relief.

In March of 1997, Sharon had a complete physical examination that included a mammogram. The day following the exam her doctor called to say that they had seen something suspicious in the mammogram and that surgery was required to determine exactly what it was.

Sharon went into a hospital the following week for a lumpectomy. Two days following the surgery Sharon was told she had breast cancer. She and Ed were shocked. They consulted with a cancer specialist who confirmed the diagnosis.

Sharon's doctor told her that her cancer was localized and there was no indication that the cancer had spread to any surrounding tissue or to her lymph system.

Three separate doctors recommended additional surgery to either clean out the area or to remove the breast completely. A daily six week course of radiation treatment was also recommended.

Sharon and Ed nearly caved into the terror of cancer. But they called me to see what I had to say. I explained to them that cancer was an indication of a failing immune system. Lumps, etc. show up locally, but

73

the problem is systemic which indicates an entirely toxic body. If the symptoms are treated or removed and the problem is not solved, the symptoms will simply pop up again somewhere else in the body. This is why women, in as little as six months after surgery, show up with symptoms in other parts of there body, even after they were told by their doctors that they had "gotten it all."

I told them about my friend Lucianna. She was told that her cancer was localized. Lucianna was filled with fear and opted to have her breast removed — the *symptom* removed — and then undergo the radiation treatment. Her doctors said they "got it all" — two years later the cancer spread and there was nothing they could then do, except once again try to treat the symptoms. She died.

I also explained to Sharon and Ed that cancer cells are nothing more than abnormal cells. We all get them now and then. But a healthy immune system cleans them up before they get out of control. Cancer is never a localized disease. *Get that straight.* And the usual treatments for it are unnatural and totally illogical. That's why they fail.

Sharon's immune system was compromised. Her "never getting sick" actually meant that her body was never cleaning house. It was storing poisons and not eliminating them. After years and years of poisoning her body, her immune system gave up and she got hit all at once.

Sharon and Ed began to consider various alternative way of dealing with the cancer. Of course they were bombarded by their family and friends, who spoke up out of genuine concern and love, but also out of ignorance.

After long talks and much consideration, Sharon decided not to have the surgery or the radiation treatments. She opted instead to strengthen her immune system and allow her own body to rid itself of the cancer cells.

Sharon began a strict juice diet, drinking only freshly squeezed (never bottled) organic citrus fruits such as oranges, grapefruits, tangelos and also some juiced tomatoes. She drank as much as she wanted, whenever she wanted — usually about 96 ounces a day. This continued for 50 days.

About the second week on juice, Sharon realized that her menopause symptoms had completely vanished. The night sweats and hot flashes had stopped and her mood swings had ceased. Sharon said she also had an "improved sense of well being."

After three weeks on juice, Sharon's shoulder pain had completely stopped and her grip strength had returned. She also noticed that her energy level was much higher than before — higher then she could ever remember.

Sharon's lifestyle has completely changed as a result of her cancer scare. She still drinks a lot of fresh, organic juices and she eats fruits and some veggies — all organic and raw. Sharon vows that she will never return to her old eating habits. She loves her new body — she's lean and fit with lots of energy. Now, without the menopause symptoms and the shoulder pain, she has renewed sexual energy. She and Ed are finally enjoying their lives.

Sharon knows that her immune system is working. She and Ed know that the cancer is gone but I asked her to go back to the doctor so the rest of the world could have medical *proof*.

On July 1, 1997, Sharon and Ed returned for a medical opinion. After examining Sharon and talking with her and Ed, the doctor said, "Don't tell my other patients what you're doing — it will put me out of business."

On July 29, 1997, her mammogram was negative — no sign of cancer.

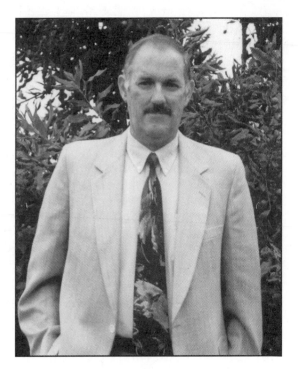

Bob

Bob

Bob was diagnosed in 1992 with Chronic Lymphocytic Leukemia (CCL) at the age of 47. His doctors said his aliment normally appears in older people, not somebody his age. They couldn't trace it to any particular reason. With the exception of one brother, there is no cancer in his entire family.

They told Bob that a bone marrow transplant was the only possible medical cure for the disease, however, they recommended the procedure only as a last resort. Bone marrow transplants are used as a last resort because the high level of radiation treatment and chemotherapy that is needed to kill off all the white blood cells could also kill off the immune system.

However, chemotherapy became the treatment of choice. Are low doses safe? Or are they killing the immune system slowly?

Before Bob started his first treatment his white blood count had elevated to about 65,000. The normal range is 9,000 to 10,000. Less than one-third of his white cells were normal.

Bob's first treatment lasted seven months and consisted of taking 44 pills during one day of each month. They told him that this high dosage, intermittent treatment, was to blast the cells and then allow the system to purge itself during the rest of the month. He had nausea and fatigue which lasted about three days after the treatment and became more intense after each month. His white blood count gradually decreased to about 15,000 but the ratio of his normal white cells was still less than half.

Because they treated the symptoms instead of addressing the problem, Bob's white cell count was back to 45,000 within two years. The medical solution for this was to give a different and stronger drug and to give more of it. They administered his new chemotherapy drug intravenously in one hour sessions for five consecutive days each month for five months. His white cell count went down to 13,000.

This time it only took a year and a half before his white cell count was high again. In March of 1997, his count was 30,000 and climbing. In April of 1997, another chemotherapy session was ordered. This is when I met Bob. I explained about how the immune system works and his chances of surviving yet another chemotherapy treatment were not good. Bob knew he wasn't getting better, so he decided to work on ridding his body of toxins and building up his immune system.

He started on fresh organic fruit and juice on May 2, 1997. After about three weeks into this program his skin started to get worse. His face, neck, chest and back broke out in large pus-filled eruptions. He was miserable. I was thrilled. When I explained to Bob that his body was dumping the poison in his blood stream out through the largest elimination organ — the skin, he was thrilled too. I told him not to put anything on his skin except water.

Bob lost weight and gained energy.

On July 2, 1997, he went in for another blood test. Bob called me as soon as he finished with the doctor. His white blood count dropped to 24,000. His doctor was amazed and told him he was "actually getting better." In the five years since his diagnosis, his white blood count had never dropped without massive chemotherapy. Bob said, "I was a three-quarter believer when we started but now I believe 100%."

Stephanie

I met Stephanie almost two years ago when she hired me as her health and fitness coach. She is a successful attorney with a private practice in San Francisco. Cute, petite and ready for anything, Stephanie was fit already but she wanted more. She wanted more energy, more stamina and a really tight body. She thought that normal aging was slowing her down, but after meeting me, she threw out that idea completely — Stephanie and I are the same age.

I put her on an exercise program and she started to make some changes in her diet, adding more fresh organic fruits and vegetables. The program worked very well for her. She had more energy and her body was looking great.

We worked together for about a year. Then, in early August, 1996, she started having occasional dizzy spells. She would feel fine all day, fall asleep at a normal time, then wake up about an hour later feeling extremely weak, nauseated and dizzy. She also suffered occasional ear aches, hoarseness and had a consistent low grade fever. I wanted to put her on a fast to clean her out. She said absolutely no! She was going to seek medical advice. She liked me, but after all, I wasn't a doctor.

The first doctor she consulted suspected a low thyroid problem. He ordered a thyroid test, which came back normal. In spite of the normal results, he strongly recommended she take Synthroid, a drug that was given to people with low thyroid problems. After several days on the Synthroid, she became sicker than ever. I voiced my disagreement about her taking the drug and pushed her, once again, to consider a fast. She flatly refused, thinking I was crazy — after all, she just might have a thyroid problem.

In August 1996, her eight month nightmare began. The dizzy spells began hitting at all times of the day and night. She became highly susceptible to episodes of extreme anxiety and panic attacks. She ended up in the hospital emergency room on several different occasions and was finally referred to a neurologist. The neurologist suspected multiple sclerosis or myasthenia gravis or a brain tumor and ordered an MRI. She was an emotional wreck, as you can imagine. After almost three weeks of thinking the worst, they finally had the

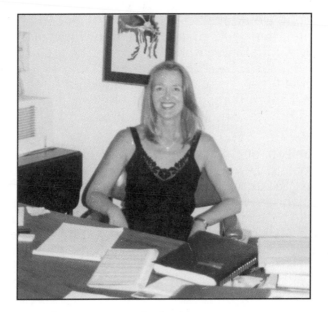

Stephanie

MRI and it was normal. The neurologist gave her a vague diagnosis of labyrinthitis, which is an infection of the inner ear and told her she "had to live with it," but that it would probably get better. He advised her to take Antivert (a drug for dizziness). She decided to consult with an ear specialist, who agreed with the neurologist's diagnosis.

Last January she took a trip to Sedona, Arizona with her boyfriend, David. She still hadn't been feeling very well but the dizzy spells were fairly under control and she assumed she was on the mend. By the time they reached Sedona, three days after leaving San Francisco, she was so ill she could hardly stand up by herself. On her fourth day there, she ended up back in the hospital emergency room in Flagstaff. The doctors told her it was probably the labyrinthitis being aggravated by the higher local altitude. They prescribed more Antivert and added Valium for the anxiety. They told her she'd feel better once she got back to sea level.

Back in San Francisco, she consulted the ear specialist as well as the neurologist she had previously seen. They both told her they weren't really sure what was going on but that she would have to live with the problem. She continued to occasionally take the Antivert and Valium.

Two weeks later she became so ill that she literally could not get from her bed to the bathroom without assistance. She began to have trouble focusing her eyes. Reading became impossible. She had to stop wearing her contact lenses because focusing on anything made her feel extremely ill. She couldn't comfortably move her head or her eyes. An acquaintance told her that his mother had the same problem and that she'd had to give up driving. She became extremely depressed and stopped eating. Her sister flew in from Chicago to help care for her. She ended up in her general practitioner's office, this time feeling that if she didn't get some relief she would actually die from malnutrition before anything else. Her doctor hospitalized her.

While she was in the hospital, the doctors increased her Antivert prescription and switched her from Valium to Xanax. She became addicted to the Xanax. They took an MRI of her gastrointestinal tract because they suspected she had a pancreatic tumor. She didn't. A psychiatrist switched her back to the Valium and recommended Zoloft for her anxiety. She took two doses of the Zoloft and got even sicker. On her tenth day in the hospital, her nurse confided in her that she felt she needed "an alternative approach." The nurse performed accupressure on her head and for the first time Stephanie began to feel some relief.

That night David called me and told me what had happened. He said he wanted to take her out of the hospital and asked me if I would see her. David checked Stephanie out of the hospital the following morning and I saw her that afternoon.

After examining Stephanie, I told her she probably had an inner ear infection. This was causing the dizziness and the low-grade fever. Stephanie said that the nurse that did the accupressure told her the same thing. Stephanie could not move her eyes from side to side without passing out. She was heavily drugged. She couldn't stand up without assistance and she definitely couldn't walk. I gave her a cranial treatment and she relaxed. David said they were committed to doing whatever I suggested. Stephanie wanted me to help her.

David and Stephanie had begun to believe that I had been right all along. Immediately, Stephanie stopped taking the medication and started drinking pure, fresh, organic orange juice. Stephanie was not on the medication long enough, as Ed had been, so the "cold turkey" approach was not life threatening.

The first week Stephanie went through hell. She was detoxing off the medications and she was terribly frightened. My program challenged all of her beliefs. What she was doing was going against everything the experts told her. Plus, she was physically, as well as emotionally, exhausted, to put it mildly. Stephanie and I talked at least five or six times a day and sometimes more. She needed loads of emotional support.

The fourth night of drinking only juice was the worst. She was awake all night, writhing, shaking, crying and praying. The next morning she started to calm down. She was extremely weak but the shaking had stopped.

Stephanie continued on the juice only program for three more days. She was still extremely frightened. I knew we had to get the drugs and the infection out even faster, so I took her to my home for a water fast. During a water fast, the body can devote even more of its energy and focus to cleansing — because it doesn't even have the juice to work on digesting. It only took three days on water to see some incredible changes. The next day I took her back to her home, put her back on the juice only program and started her on a light exercise program of walking and stretching. She started wearing her contacts again and was able to read just fine.

On the eleventh day after checking out of the hospital she was driving again. I went over to her house in my little sports car, put the top down, put her behind the wheel and she drove us all over town — no problem. She almost cried.

Stephanie now thrives on fresh organic fruit and some veggies. She went back to her doctor to get his reaction. He couldn't believe the change. He called her experience a "quest." He admitted that he knew she had been dying and that he didn't know how to get her better. He said: "The fast was a great idea — it saved your life."

One day, as I was leaving Stephanie's house, David said, "You know, Roe, I used to have a healthy skepticism for the medical profession. Now I'm totally paranoid."

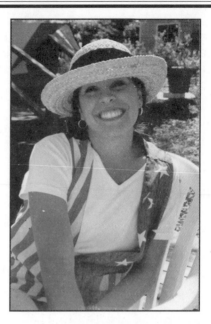

Sonia and Fouad

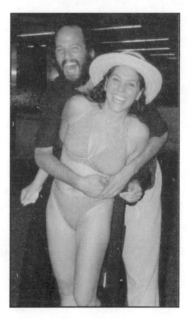

Sonia

Sonia had been on a vegan diet, 75 percent raw food diet before going on a five month trip to several Central American countries. The first two months she managed to stay on her diet. After two months she began eating rice and beans, then even fried bananas, bread, coffee, cheese and finally chocolate. She stopped exercising and refused to get on a scale or look into a full length mirror.

We saw each other two days after she got home. She said I looked radiant, that my eyes were clear and that my body was still petite and as strong as hers had been before she left. She saw how much energy I had and she cried. She didn't know how she could have let herself get to be 25 pounds overweight, tired, lazy and fat. Her self-image was, of course, extremely low. She expected me to lecture her, but instead I asked: "Well, did you enjoy eating all that food? Was it good?" She looked at me and then we both laughed hysterically. I encouraged her to do a juice fast and promised to do it with her. She reluctantly began juicing the following day but she didn't feel ready. She ended the fast.

Several weeks later she met the authors of *Natures First Law* and found their book extremely motivating. A few days later she approached me again, now wanting to do a juice fast. Again, I agreed to do it with her. This time she was committed. She wanted to drop those pounds and restore her energy. She drank only fresh squeezed juice for 40 days — from two to four 32 oz. glasses of orange, tangerine or grapefruit juice each day. The first few days were difficult because she felt exhausted, cranky and depressed. Her face broke out in small pimples, she sneezed a lot and had three very painful canker sores in her mouth. After the third week her skin was clear, soft and supple. She had suffered from acne since she was a teenager and this was the first time her skin had actually been clear. Her eyes were bright. She even noticed that some scars and undiagnosed lumps beginning to disappear. Her negative emotions of depression, anger and crankiness were replaced with loving thoughts and feelings. She radiated these feelings and people immediately responded.

Sonia learned quickly that what she ate became either energy or poison. She was back on track and looking and feeling great with clear skin, a lean and fit body and lots of energy.

"I'm a true believer in fasting," she now says. "If you are considering fasting to improve your health or clean out your body, I strongly suggest that you do it. If it's your first time, I suggest that you have your fast monitored by someone like Roe, who can offer you their knowledge, advice and support."

David

David is not a client of mine but he is one of my dear friends. I know his story will help others.

David was already well on the path of health when I met him. But that wasn't always the case.

As a teen, David was always fit and seemingly healthy despite eating meat, bread and junk food. However, at age 17, his robust energy began to gradually decline. David's physical and mental energies deteriorated over a period of six months, then he experienced incessant diarrhea. After a few weeks of medicine treatment, he showed little improvement, so a colon examination was done. The diagnosis was ulcerative colitis. He spent his 18th birthday in a hospital, taking prednisone and Azulfadine drug treatments. The symptoms subsided temporarily, but the drugs further ruined his health.

Within a few months after the hospital stay, still feeling sickly and very weak, he experienced a recurrence of the diarrhea and additional symptoms, including cramping and bleeding. This lead to further physical deterioration. The following eight years were filled with colitis flare-ups chronic fatigue and off-and-on drug therapy. During this time, David struggled through engineering school then three years of environmental engineering employment. At age 26, David was reduced to a weak, sickly shadow of his former self. He was having gastric explosions every time he ate and up to 10 painful bowel movements a day with mucus and blood. His nervous system was shattered. He was toxic — debilitated by the medicines and severely demineralized.

Life had become a dying hell for David. He never gave in to the medical doctors' advice to accept his illness and just be patient until the "miracle drug cure" came along. David desperately wanted his health back and doubted that the doctors knew what they were doing.

In 1984, David had the great fortune to find a doctor of Natural Hygiene, Laurence Galant, in Staten Island. Dr. Galant introduced him to the concepts of self-healing and eating a raw fruit-based diet. At first, David thought the idea of eating mostly fruit while he was having non-stop diarrhea was crazy. He studied Natural Hygiene and slowly started to clean up his diet but he was still attached to eating chicken and other favorite foods and was still relying on medicines and still having colitis flare-ups.

In the fall of 1984, David had a colonoscopy exam which confirmed that he had advanced ulcerations throughout his colon. Assuming that he had been chronically sick and was not getting better, the gastroenterologist recommended that David either try his experimental drug, 6-mercaptopurine, which knocks out the immune system (some doctors believe that the immune system causes colitis) or have his colon surgically removed. Upon hearing that, a heavy decisive thought entered David's mind: *The doctor's advice is insane!*

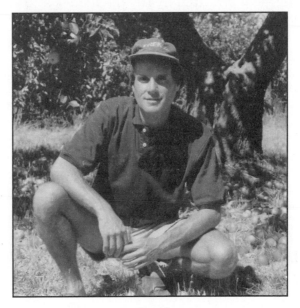

David

David had had it with the medical madness. He thought that he would soon be dead unless he found the answer for himself. David recognized that his life was a gradual descent into hell. He knew that it was now time to climb out or it would be too late.

Over the next few days, David started thinking critically about how to overcome his illness He considered more closely the information on self-healing and raw food eating. Finally, it made sense. David naturally decided to change to a fruit-based diet knowing he was going to heal.

The next day David threw away the medicine, gave up all meat and dairy and started a three-day juice cleanse. By the second day, he was coming back to life. On the third day, he was feeling so much better and exuding so much joy that his enthusiasm drove his family and friends crazy! His gut was soothed and he was starting to rejuvenate. His digestion became perfect. His stools became formed and his bowel movements became easy. David's colon completely healed up within six weeks. He set himself free of illness, doctors and medicine for good.

David adopted a diet of about 90% fruit. His energy continuously increased as he detoxified and began rebuilding his depleted body.

I met David in 1994, just after he left engineering to become a certified Nutrition Educator. Since 1994, he has provided nutrition and health consultations based on his knowledge and his experience. David is a living example of what he teaches. David also publishes *Living Nutrition*, a magazine he created for health education. He owns and operates the Living Nutrition Guidance Center in Sebastopol, California, and he also directs Colitis and Ileitis Health Education Services.

For David, his 100% raw food diet of 90% fruit is not difficult at all. David says, "Living healthfully is the easiest and most joyful way to be. Euphoric health is our natural birthright."

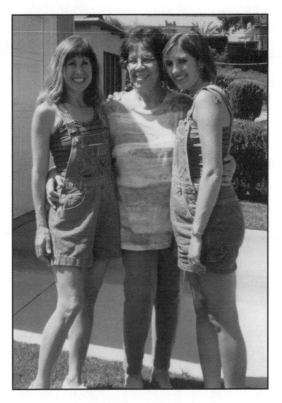

Roe, Mae and Deanna

Mae

Mae is a powerful example of how you can get healthy at any age. Mae lived on a standard American diet all of her life and suffered 30 years from allergies, upper respiratory infections and high blood pressure. In spite of seeking and receiving prompt medications and treatment from her doctors, her blood pressure continued to climb. In April of 1984, Mae's blood pressure peaked at 240/130. During this time her temperature rose to 105 degrees and stayed there for five days. She was diagnosed with a viral infection and an infection in her left kidney. Also, her hemoglobin was 8.0g/dl. A healthy hemoglobin count is about 15g/dl.

Mae was hospitalized for 17 days and given a myriad of treatments and medications. Besides the many drugs for infection, she was given Allopurinol for gout, Atenolol and Hydralazine for high blood pressure, Acetaminophen (analgesic for fever) with Codeine (for pain), Meperidine and Demerol, both narcotics for pain, Fergon, an iron supplement for anemia and Compazine and Flurazepam, both tranquilizers to get her through this wretched experience.

Her immune system was not able to keep up with the amount of poison her body was consuming on a regular basis. Over the next 13 years her blood pressure stayed high, although she was still taking even more medication. She experienced frequent infections, especially ear infections until she lost 50% of her hearing in both of her ears. She had constant bouts with sinus infections, headaches and constipation. Her vision deteriorated, her skin started to lose pigment and dry out and her hair also became dry and started falling out. Mae developed painful arthritis and experienced sore and weak muscles. She also developed more environmental allergies and chronic bronchitis. She also gained weight. These symptoms were not signs of aging as she was lead to believe. Her body was reacting to the poison she was taking in through her medication and her food.

In April of 1997, her blood pressure continued to increase and her blood pressure meds were not working. She was taking Maxidex, a steroid for her allergies; Traimterene, a diuretic for water retention, Clonidine, Lotensin and Atenolol for high blood pressure, Lodine, and anti-inflammatory for arthritis. Last but not least, Paxil for her depression.

Her niece, Brenda, asked me to call her. I met with Mae in May of 1997 and went over her history. Mae was a toxic waste dump and she knew it. Her blood pressure was out of control along with the rest of her body.

Mae started right away. She felt she had no time to waste. Mae started drinking fresh organic orange juice and eating some fruit and slowly started weaning herself of all her medication. In one month, her blood pressure, without medication, was down to 120/60 with a heart rate of 53. She lost 20 pounds and the arthritis and constipation were gone and so was all her medication. She is walking again and even though she still has some pain in her legs and buttocks, she walks a little more every day with a little less pain. Mae says, "You have shown and proven to me that by fasting and cleaning out my body, my health problems including high blood pressure, arthritis and constipation have disappeared without using any medication and my body is getting better."

Mae is 72 years young.

Three Ways To Create A New Belief

♦Write it

♦Say it

♦Visualize it

Write It

Proclaim your new belief by writing it down. Write it in present tense as if it is already your belief. Make sure it is a positive statement — negatives don't work. Writing your new belief creates a picture. Once you see that picture, you'll start to believe it. And once you believe it, you'll own it.

Write your new belief on index cards, post-its, anything that you can take with you. Also, hang it up on your bathroom mirror, at your desk, everywhere and anywhere. Here's an example:

I am in total control of my body. I control what I put into my mouth, so I eat fresh, organic, fruit. I control how I use my body, so I exercise at least 30 minutes a day. I control what I put into my mind, so my thoughts are positive and loving. I control who I associate with, so I surround myself with positive, loving and supportive people. I control what I do, so my work and play time is happy and productive.

Say It

You talk to yourself all the time. Do you pay attention to what you say? Do you say, "I'm so stupid, why did I do that?" or, "That's not like me, I can do better?" Do you tell yourself, "I'm great," or, "I'm an idiot?" What you tell yourself is what you become. You move in the direction of your most currently dominant thought. Do you say "I'm in control of my life" or "I'll never be able to do it, it's too hard?" If you tell yourself you're in control, then you will be in control. If you tell yourself something is too hard, then it will be too hard for you and you'll fail.

Say your new belief out loud at least ten times a day — while you're driving, exercising or showering. The more you say it, the faster you'll believe it. And once you believe it, you'll own it.

Visualize It

What you see is what you get. Visualization is one of the major steps to creating an empowering belief and getting what you want.

Visualization creates a vivid and exact fantasy of your new belief. Use your imagination because your imagination rules your world. People have been saying this for lifetimes — and it's true.

When you use your imagination in a positive way, you anticipate success.

Dr. Dennis Waitley, who did motivational work with Olympic athletes, found that winners expect to win in advance. Top athletes are trained to imagine the end of their event and then envision themselves as winners. Then they live the winning scene over and over during practice sessions. Now, with the help of advanced technology, Olympic athletes can even see their image superimposed on a video showing them as the winner. They watch themselves win again and again until their actual performance begins. They see themselves winning. They believe they can win. They win.

What you truly imagine yourself to be is what you become. At first you won't believe your imagination. But don't let that stop you. Keep seeing yourself there. Do this over and over again and you'll believe it. And once you believe it, you'll have it.

Five Questions to Lock in a Powerful Visualization

- How will you look and feel?
- What will you say to yourself?
- How will others see you and feel about you?
- What will others say to you?
- How will this goal affect your relationships, your career — your life?

Answer these questions in detail.

Now, see yourself already there. Visualize yourself as lean, fit and healthy. Get out pictures of when you were at your desired weight. If you were never there, take a picture of you and cut out your face and put it on a picture of someone who has the body you should have. Make copies and hang them up on your refrigerator, desk and everywhere else.

What You Visualize You Can Achieve

The power of the mind is *so* strong. Thoughts are things that can materialize, so be careful to focus on what you *want*. Who you think you are and who you imagine yourself to be is what you become. You move in the direction of your most current and dominant thoughts. Your beliefs are based on information that comes into your subconscious through your five senses. Sometimes this information is positive and sometimes negative. The good news is — you don't have to live your life based on any piece of information. If positive information comes into your senses, your beliefs will be positive. But if you are bombarded with negative information — change it, make it positive. You can create positive empowering beliefs.

As a small child I had a traumatic fall: my forehead was cut open and my nose was broken and bloody. My mother, frightened and fearful, screamed, "you're so clumsy!" Because the great emotional pain accompanied intense physical pain, her critical message was deeply imprinted in my belief system. Every time I fell, this negative message was reinforced, either by my mother or by my own negative beliefs.

Each fall strengthened my belief that I was clumsy. My longing to participate in activities that required coordination, like dance, was in direct conflict with the belief I had that I was clumsy. When I thought about dancing, my subconscious took that thought and succumbed to the belief that I was clumsy. My subconscious would deliver the message: "forget it, because dancing requires a coordination you lack." Over the years I managed to change my belief of clumsiness. I kept seeing myself as an excellent dancer, graceful and fluid. Today, I *am* an excellent dancer. My programming about falling and the pain surrounding my falls, still makes me fearful of activities that require downhill balance. But I face these fears and work through more of my negative beliefs every time I put on my Roller Blades.

Visualization can help you change negative beliefs to positive ones. You can even change the affects of traumas from the past. Do this by changing your perspective on what happened (reframing) or mentally changing what happened (rescripting).

Change Negative Beliefs

♦ Reframing

♦ Rescripting

Reframing

Reframing takes a negative picture and puts a positive frame around it. Because I was so sick as a child, I had a lot of pain. Now, when I look back at my childhood, I see the same pictures of my unhealthy state, but with different frames: I see the knowledge I gained about the human body, my appreciation for health and life and my ability to empathize with others and help them get healthy.

Reframing is looking for the good in every situation, no matter how bad it seems.

Remember Sonia? When her mother suffered a massive heart attack, she called me, crying. Her mom was still alive. I told her to be thankful that her mother, at 47 years old, had this incredible warning. Some people aren't as lucky. Now her mom has the opportunity to clean out her body, get healthy and live a long and productive life — and to be able to play with her grandchildren.

Rescripting

Rescripting lets you visually change a negative scene into a positive one. For example, at nine I wanted to be on Ted Mack's Original Amateur Hour, the local TV talent scout program where I lived. I longed to perform, particularly to sing and dance with Fred Astaire. When I wrote a letter to Ted Mack expressing my desire to be on his show, my mom laughed at me and told me I was ridiculous. I wasn't discouraged by her remark but went to a store to buy some sheet music. I rehearsed everyday after school, singing my little song. The school's music teacher helped, accompanying me on the piano. I finally got a letter from Ted Mack — an invitation to audition for his show. Thrilled and excited, considering this to be my big break, I practiced and counted the days.

I was dressed in my best Sunday dress, ready to go, when my mother refused to let me. She told me I was silly and ridiculous and that it was an entirely crazy idea. I remember crying for a very long time. I felt destroyed. I can still summon up the scene as if it were yesterday.

Yet a conscious recollection of that scene wasn't always possible. I blanked it out for a long time, trapping it in my subconscious where it held me back from successfully engaging in creative dreams. One evening, before I gave my first lecture on communication, I was practicing a visualization of my anticipation of success, when suddenly I was nine years old, getting ready to go to the Ted Mack audition. It was almost 25 years later when I was finally able to recall what happened. My mom didn't mean to harm me; she feared show business and wanted to protect me. Not knowing this then, I assumed I couldn't go because I wasn't good enough. Imagine what that did to my self esteem! The experience was so traumatic; it left a deep and lasting impression on my subconscious.

The stronger the emotions are concerning an event, the more magnified the picture is in our subconscious. Negative or positive, all emotions have a direct effect on the size and impact of how we remember an event. And the more traumatic the scene, the more we tend to blank it out. Even though I hadn't remembered what had happened for a long time, I suffered the effects on my belief system. This event needed to be rescripted.

In order to rescript a scene, you play it in its original form, then play it as you want it to be, using the present tense and positive emotions. You also make sure you get the outcome you desire. The new script is played again and again until the positive picture becomes bigger than the negative one. It's good to remember that your subconscious records information without discriminating between reality or imagination.

So now when I'm asked to give a lecture, my belief system tells me that I'm going to be a success. In my rescripted scene my mom buys me a new dress and she and my dad take me to the audition. On the way to the audition my parents tell me how proud they are of me and how confident they are that I'll be great. When we get to the audition, the theater is full. When I finish my act everyone applauds and cheers. Of course, Ted Mack asks me to be on his show. My parents are ecstatic and I am happy. Since the subconscious doesn't care whether the information is real or imagined, the scene can be as outrageous as you want it to be. My audition scene ends with thousands of people screaming and clapping. My parents lead the call for an encore. This is a powerful scene I relive over and over and use every time before I do something challenging. My positive belief now far outweighs any negative programming.

Reliving successful feelings over and over, regardless of whether these feelings are real or imagined, contributes to powerful positive beliefs.

Create an empowering belief. Write it. Say it. Visualize it. Now you are ready to live it.

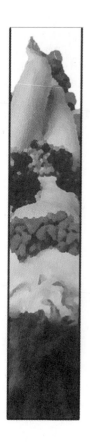

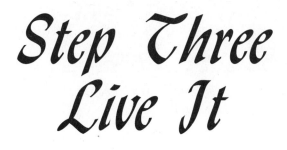

*Step Three
Live It*

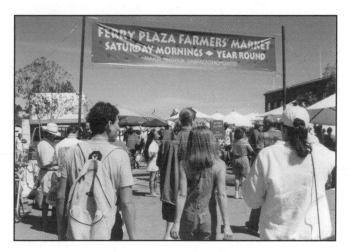

Shopping for fruit can be fun!

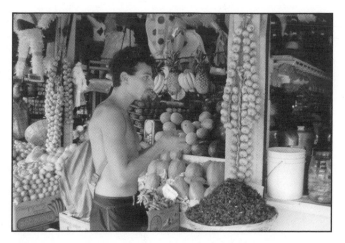

David Wolfe along with his co-authors Stephen Arlin and Fouad Dini say "...cooked food is poison..." throughout their new book "Nature's First Law"

4

STEP THREE
LIVE IT

Six Ways To Live Your Beliefs

Information isn't enough and believing it isn't enough. You must *totally* live it in order to benefit from it.

- ♦Decide
- ♦Commit
- ♦Set a goal
- ♦Make a plan
- ♦Work your plan
- ♦Be persistent

Decide

Have you tried diets and exercise programs and found that you couldn't stick to them? What went wrong?

First, you need to decide what you want. What does this mean? To decide means literally to cut off all other options. To decide to have a perfect body means not settling for anything less and not stopping the process until you accomplish your goal. This decision is a life or death decision that will permanently affect the quality of your life — every minute of it! I made a conscious decision to get healthy and nothing or no one was going to stand in the way of that decision. I didn't have a choice. Do you? Decide now!

Commit

What is commitment? Imagine a small boy trapped at the bottom of a 100 foot drop. You are at the top looking down and no one else is available to help rescue him. There is a rope next to you and it is long enough to reach the child. You make a small lasso and lower it down to him. You instruct the child to put the lasso around his chest. You start to pull. You have to go very slowly because the side of the cliff is very jagged. If you pull too quickly you could severely hurt or kill him. Half way up, it starts to rain. You're wet, cold and tired. What do you do? Do you drop the rope because it's too difficult to keep pulling and let the child die? No, you continue. *This is commitment!* Never give up. Hold on to that rope. Real commitment transcends the impossible. It is so rewarding it becomes a joy.

People who are determined take responsibility for getting what they want. Have you noticed that people who are not successful usually blame something or someone outside themselves for their failures (the government, their boss, their family background); whereas people who are successful often have similar obstacles but take the responsibility for overcoming them. Having determination means not deviating from your goals, being laser-focused. Being laser-focused means concentrating on your goal and being willing to do whatever it takes to achieve it.

When you say, "I've tried to change my eating habits but it just didn't work for me" or "I have a hard time locating organic produce where I live," were you committed? Were you determined? I don't think so! What has stopped you, in the past, from really committing?

What happens if you fall — does this mean you're not committed? No. It just means you fell. When you're really committed you pick yourself up and keep on going. Making mistakes and giving into old negative programming is not failure — giving up is. Write down all your prior excuses, justifications and negative programming. Then write out this statement:

Commitment means holding onto the rope, placing one hand over the other until the child is safe. Commitment is being willing to do whatever it takes. Commitment is my word, my honor, my integrity, my success.

Set A Goal

Once you have decided and committed you are ready to make a plan and put it into action. Before you write your daily plan, write out your goal. This statement should contain the three P's: it should be powerful, positive and in present tense.

Here's an example that I wrote for a client of mine. When we started working together, about a year ago, she weighed 303 pounds. She now weighs 200 pounds and the weight keeps coming off. These words are now her's:

I lost 173 pounds. Because I am five feet, eight inches, at 130 pounds I look fabulous. My legs are long and shapely and my stomach is flat. I have a lot of energy to do whatever I want. My blood pressure is low and my health is excellent. I feel unstoppable.

Every time I get dressed and look in the mirror I say, 'Damn,

I look good.' After an effortless climb up several flights of stairs I say, 'I am soooo fit.'

Other people look at me in amazement. People who don't know me think I'm gorgeous and people who do know me think I'm amazing for accomplishing such an incredible undertaking. My husband thinks I'm superwoman.

My friends and family keep saying, 'You did it, you really did it and you look fabulous. You're an inspiration.' People who don't know me say, 'You're in such great shape, it must be genetic.'

My husband and I have more fun because I'm confident, playful and have tons of energy. I love myself so much that I can love him even more. My incredible self-love has made me more loving, empathetic and compassionate to all people and my self-esteem, self-confidence and self-worth give me unstoppable personal power which positively affects my career both with money and recognition.

See how detailed this goal statement is? Being specific is very crucial to getting what you want.

Make A Plan

Your plan needs to be detailed. Your plan must elaborate exactly what you will do on a day to day basis to reach your goal. Here's an outline:

♦ Entertain only positive, loving thoughts.

♦ Eat mostly fresh organic fruits.

♦ Exercise for a least 30 minutes a day.

When you follow this outline, you will be healthy, both in mind and body and you will attract love and success.

Write down a step-by-step daily plan. Make it as detailed as possible.

Also, write how you're feeling, both physically and emotionally. It's important to record your feelings during this time of change. When you write out your feelings you learn a lot about why you do what you do. Especially when it comes to old, bad habits.

Work Your Plan

This is your final action step. You have all the information, new beliefs and a plan on how to get there. Now it's time to *just do it*.

Example:

♦ Think wonderful, loving and supportive thoughts toward yourself and others. Make these your beliefs. Reinforce your positive beliefs by visualizing them, writing them in a journal and affirming them out loud. Seek guidance and encouragement and surround yourself with positive, supportive people.

♦ Choose and eat only a small amount of fresh, raw, organic fruits. Lay out your food for the day. Eat only what is on your daily plan and nothing more!

♦ Exercise at least 30 minutes a day. Do aerobic and strength training exercises. Measure your accomplishments and compare them to your goals.

Be Persistent

Sometimes being persistent isn't easy — just ask my friend Lisa. Don't give up no matter how many times you seem to fail. Remember Thomas Edison — he failed more than 10,000 times before he succeeded in creating the light bulb. Abraham Lincoln won the Presidency but he had no formal education and had previously lost so many political elections that people laughed at him for continuing to try. In 1962, Decca Records rejected The Beetles, telling them that guitar music was on its

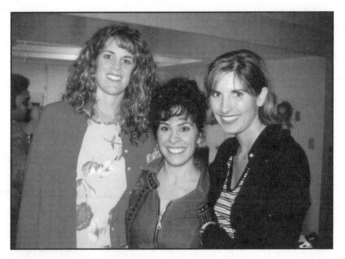

Lisa joined Sonia and Deanna on their quest for health. Lisa, the six foot tall beauty got rid of her migraines because she was persistant. She says, "I never had so much energy or felt so healthy. I feel more alert — all my senses seem to be more improved. It's a new me."

way out. Steve Jobs was rejected by both Atari and Hewlett-Packard before he went on to build Apple Computer. Fred Smith got a "C" grade from his Yale University Management Professor on his paper proposing overnight delivery service. His professor said the concept was interesting but in order to earn better than a "C" the idea must be feasible. Fred Smith went on to found Federal Express.

These are examples of people who didn't give up. I didn't give up and neither did my clients and friends and now we've regained our health after modern medicine gave up on us. Don't *you* give up.

So live it. Start right now on your daily journal and decide, commit, set a goal, make a plan, work your plan and be persistent.

Take Charge

Follow these three steps for your perfect body — get it, believe it and live it.

Do this and you'll be on top of the world — healthy, happy and full of energy.

Take charge of your life, right now and thrive. Have that perfect body no matter how old you are. Decide what you want — visualize it, believe it and make it a reality. With a pure-cleaned-out body and mind you're headed for success.

Your new lifestyle will give you the energy you need to really enjoy everything. You'll get better as you get older. I know this is true. Make the decision to be lean, fit and healthy for the rest of your life. Make this decision, today. Believe you can do it and you will. You'll look and feel incredible, have radiant health, tons of energy and lots of fun. You'll have a perfect body.

I Breathe

They don't understand.
They are confused.
Forgive them —
They don't know what they are doing.
They mean no harm.
Their vision is narrow.
Their intention is good.
Still the pain moves through my body.
I feel their pain.
I sense their agony.
I can see their death.
How do I lead them from the pain?
I can't.
What do I say to them to make them hear?
Nothing.
I am mute.
I am expressionless.
I breathe.

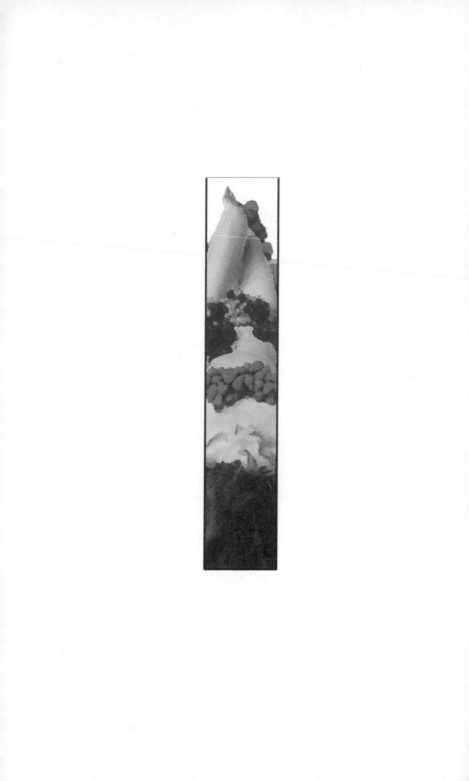

Perfect Body
Journal

Notes

Decide

Decide now and cut off all other possibilities. Read this statement ten times with resolve then sign it.

I have decided to take 100 percent responsibility for my body. I have decided to have a perfect body, a body that is lean, fit and healthy and nothing will stop me from accomplishing my goal. I know that this decision will affect the quality of my life; every minute of it.

Signature: _____

Date: _____

Notes

Commit

Commit to yourself. Read this commitment ten times, with determination, and sign it.

I am 100 percent committed to being lean, fit, and healthy.

I am 100 percent committed to having unstoppable energy and radiant health.

I am 100 percent committed to being disease and pain free.

Signature:_____

Date:_____

Notes

Set Your Goal

Take the time right now to write your goal statement. Read it at least 10 times with excitement then sign it.

Go back to Chapter Four and look at the example under goal setting. Make sure it is includes the three P's—present tense, positive and powerful. Make it as detailed as possible.

Write out your goal NOW!

Goal Statement:

Signature: _____

Date: _____

Notes

Beliefs

Use the following positive and powerful belief or create your own, sign it and own it. Next, write your belief on anything that you can carry around with you. Post it on your bathroom mirror, refrigerator, over your desk—everywhere and anywhere. Say this belief over and over during the course of your day, at least 10 times, with conviction.

I am in total control of my body. I control what I put into my mouth, so I eat fresh, organic fruit. I control how I use my body, so I exercise and stretch all my muscles every day. I control what I put into my mind, so my thoughts are positive and loving. I control who I associate with, so I surround myself with positive, loving and supportive people. I control what I do, so my work and play time is happy and productive.

Signature: _____

Date: _____

Notes

New Beliefs

List the Disadvantages of *not* Believing it.

What are your old beliefs costing you?

List 10 disadvantages of not changing your beliefs.

1.

2.

3.

4.

5.

6.

7.

8.

9.

10.

Notes

New Beliefs

List the Advantages of Believing it

How will this new belief benefit you?

List 10 advantages of changing your beliefs.

1.

2.

3.

4.

5.

6.

7.

8.

9.

10.

Notes

Visualize

What you imagine yourself to be is what you tend to become.

Answer these five question, in detail, to lock in a powerful visualization. Write out your answers then see yourself there.

1. How will I look and feel?

2. What will I say to myself?

3. How will others see me and feel about me?

4. What will others say to me?

5. How will this goal affect my relationships, career and my life?

Notes

Visualize

Get out pictures, right now, of when you were at your perfect weight. If you were never there, take a picture of you and cut out your face and put it on a picture of someone who has the body you should have.

Go through magazines. Find someone with your *basic body type* who has a beautiful body.

Basic body type is important. For example, if you're 5'3" and small framed don't compare yourself with someone who is 5'9" and large framed.

Put a picture here in your journal. You can also hang one up on the refrigerator or over your desk.

What I Visualize, I Can Achieve

Say this statement over and over during the course of your day, at least 10 times, with conviction.

Notes

Visualize

WHAT I VISUALIZE
I CAN ACHIEVE

(place your picture here)

Notes

Plan

Your plan needs to include three points: Be positive, eat healthy and exercise daily.

Write out 5 ways to accomplish each of these three points. I'll give you two and you fill in the rest.

Be positive.

List how you will accomplish this on a day-to-day basis.

1. Write out a positive thought for the day. Say it at least 10 times. Carry it with you. Hang it up.

2. Call someone who you know is in need and be loving and supportive. Giving is receiving.

3.

4.

5.

Notes

Plan

Eat healthy.

List how you will accomplish this on a day-to-day basis.

1. Clean out your kitchen. Get rid of everything that is not fresh, organic fruit.

2. Write down everything you eat and drink.

3.

4.

5.

Notes

Plan

Exercise daily.

List how you will accomplish this on a day-to-day basis.

Make agreements with yourself.

1. Make an agreement with yourself that you cannot get out of bed until you stretch your entire body. This should only take 10 minutes.

2. Make an agreement with yourself that you cannot eat or drink anything until you do crunches, pelvic tilts and push-ups. This should take less than 10 minutes.

3.

4.

5.

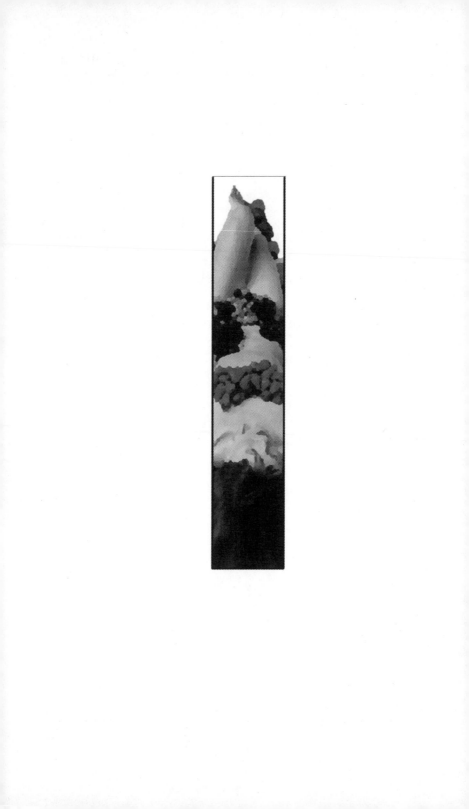

Daily Log

Daily Check List

♦ Stretch all your muscles.

♦ Read your new belief at least 10 times.

♦ Write out a positive thought for the day. Say it at least 10 times. Post it.

♦ Decide who you are going to call or visit that needs some support. Write down the person's name and phone number in your journal.

♦ Write down what you want to eat for the day.

♦ Look at your perfect body picture and visualize yourself there.

♦ Read your goal statement at least once.

♦ Do at least 30 minutes of aerobic exercise.

♦ Do the exercises in *Perfect Body*.

♦ Get rest, fresh air and sunshine.

♦ Sun your eyes for at least 10 minutes.

♦ Eat fresh, organic, seasonal, ripe fruit.

♦ Brush your teeth and tongue at least twice a day and especially before you go to bed.

♦ Floss your teeth before you go to bed.

♦ Clean your skin and your hair with warm to hot water and a cool rinse.

♦ Use a natural shampoo on your hair when needed.

♦ Clean your nails and cuticles with a nail brush.

♦ Smile often.

Daily Log Example

Thought for the Day: If I can think it, I can achieve it.

I will call and give support to: Aunt Mae (123)-123-4567

Food Log: (all fresh and organic)

64 oz. orange juice

2 apples

1 avocado

2 bananas

Exercise Log:

Stretched, 10 minutes. Walked, 30 minutes. Kick boxing class, 60 minutes. Crunches and pelvic tilts, 100 each. Squats, lunges, and side lunges, 25 each. 10 push-ups.

Skin care: Hot shower, finished with cool water. Sun and fresh air for 60 minutes.

Eye care: Sunned eyes for 10 minutes. Rested in blackness.

Hair care: Brushed hair 50 strokes. Washed with water in shower.

Nail care: Brushed nails and cuticles in shower.

Oral hygiene: Brushed teeth and tongue, morning and evening. Flossed in the evening.

Notes

Daily Journal — Day One

Be persistent. It takes about 21 days to acquire a good habit.

Thought for the Day:

I will call and give support to:

Food Log:

Exercise Log:

Skin care:

Eye care:

Hair care:

Nail care:

Oral hygiene:

Notes

Daily Journal — Day Two

Be persistent. It takes about 21 days to acquire a good habit. Congratulations! You completed one day.

Thought for the Day:

I will call and give support to:

Food Log:

Exercise Log:

Skin care:

Eye care:

Hair care:

Nail care:

Oral hygiene:

Notes

Daily Journal — Day Three

Be persistent. It takes about 21 days to acquire a good habit. Congratulations! You completed two days.

Thought for the Day:

I will call and give support to:

Food Log:

Exercise Log:

Skin care:

Eye care:

Hair care:

Nail care:

Oral hygiene:

Notes

Daily Journal — Day Four

Be persistent. It takes about 21 days to acquire a good habit. Congratulations! You completed three days.

Thought for the Day:

I will call and give support to:

Food Log:

Exercise Log:

Skin care:

Eye care:

Hair care:

Nail care:

Oral hygiene:

Notes

Daily Journal — Day Five

Be persistent. It takes about 21 days to acquire a good habit. Congratulations! You completed four days.

Thought for the Day:

I will call and give support to:

Food Log:

Exercise Log:

Skin care:

Eye care:

Hair care:

Nail care:

Oral hygiene:

Notes

Daily Journal — Day Six

Be persistent. It takes about 21 days to acquire a good habit. Congratulations! You completed five days.

Thought for the Day:

I will call and give support to:

Food Log:

Exercise Log:

Skin care:

Eye care:

Hair care:

Nail care:

Oral hygiene:

Notes

Daily Journal — Day Seven

Be persistent. It takes about 21 days to acquire a good habit. Congratulations! You completed six days.

Thought for the Day:

I will call and give support to:

Food Log:

Exercise Log:

Skin care:

Eye care:

Hair care:

Nail care:

Oral hygiene:

Notes

Daily Journal — Day Eight

Be persistent. It takes about 21 days to acquire a good habit. Congratulations! You completed seven days.

Thought for the Day:

I will call and give support to:

Food Log:

Exercise Log:

Skin care:

Eye care:

Hair care:

Nail care:

Oral hygiene:

Notes

Daily Journal — Day Nine

Be persistent. It takes about 21 days to acquire a good habit. Congratulations! You completed eight days.

Thought for the Day:

I will call and give support to:

Food Log:

Exercise Log:

Skin care:

Eye care:

Hair care:

Nail care:

Oral hygiene:

Notes

Daily Journal — Day Ten

Be persistent. It takes about 21 days to acquire a good habit. Congratulations! You completed nine days.

Thought for the Day:

I will call and give support to:

Food Log:

Exercise Log:

Skin care:

Eye care:

Hair care:

Nail care:

Oral hygiene:

Notes

Daily Journal — Day Eleven

Be persistent. It takes about 21 days to acquire a good habit.
Congratulations! You completed ten days.

Thought for the Day:

I will call and give support to:

Food Log:

Exercise Log:

Skin care:

Eye care:

Hair care:

Nail care:

Oral hygiene:

Notes

Daily Journal — Day Twelve

Be persistent. It takes about 21 days to acquire a good habit. Congratulations! You completed eleven days. You are more than half way there.

Thought for the Day:

I will call and give support to:

Food Log:

Exercise Log:

Skin care:

Eye care:

Hair care:

Nail care:

Oral hygiene:

Notes

Daily Journal — Day Thirteen

Be persistent. It takes about 21 days to acquire a good habit. Congratulations! You completed twelve days.

Thought for the Day:

I will call and give support to:

Food Log:

Exercise Log:

Skin care:

Eye care:

Hair care:

Nail care:

Oral hygiene:

Notes

Daily Journal — Day Fourteen

Be persistent. It takes about 21 days to acquire a good habit. Congratulations! You completed thirteen days.

Thought for the Day:

I will call and give support to:

Food Log:

Exercise Log:

Skin care:

Eye care:

Hair care:

Nail care:

Oral hygiene:

Notes

Daily Journal — Day Fifteen

Be persistent. It takes about 21 days to acquire a good habit. Congratulations! You completed fourteen days.

Thought for the Day:

I will call and give support to:

Food Log:

Exercise Log:

Skin care:

Eye care:

Hair care:

Nail care:

Oral hygiene:

Notes

Daily Journal — Day Sixteen

Be persistent. It takes about 21 days to acquire a good habit. Congratulations! You completed fifteen days.

Thought for the Day:

I will call and give support to:

Food Log:

Exercise Log:

Skin care:

Eye care:

Hair care:

Nail care:

Oral hygiene:

Notes

Daily Journal — Day Seventeen

Be persistent. It takes about 21 days to acquire a good habit. Congratulations! You completed sixteen days.

Thought for the Day:

I will call and give support to:

Food Log:

Exercise Log:

Skin care:

Eye care:

Hair care:

Nail care:

Oral hygiene:

Notes

Daily Journal — Day Eighteen

Be persistent. It takes about 21 days to acquire a good habit. Congratulations! You completed seventeen days.

Thought for the Day:

I will call and give support to:

Food Log:

Exercise Log:

Skin care:

Eye care:

Hair care:

Nail care:

Oral hygiene:

Notes

Daily Journal — Day Nineteen

Be persistent. It takes about 21 days to acquire a good habit. Congratulations! You completed eighteen days.

Thought for the Day:

I will call and give support to:

Food Log:

Exercise Log:

Skin care:

Eye care:

Hair care:

Nail care:

Oral hygiene:

Notes

Daily Journal — Day Twenty

Be persistent. It takes about 21 days to acquire a good habit. Congratulations! You completed nineteen days.

Thought for the Day:

I will call and give support to:

Food Log:

Exercise Log:

Skin care:

Eye care:

Hair care:

Nail care:

Oral hygiene:

Notes

Daily Journal — Day Twenty-one

Congratulations! You made it. This is your last day.

Thought for the Day:

I will call and give support to:

Food Log:

Exercise Log:

Skin care:

Eye care:

Hair care:

Nail care:

Oral hygiene:

Notes

Notes

Notes

Follow-up
Questions

Did you follow the entire 21 day plan? Describe how you feel (physically, as well as emotionally) about sticking to it or not sticking to it.

Describe your current level of commitment to your health.

Do you feel like your behavior and lifestyle is congruent with your level of commitment?

How has your current level of awareness changed regarding health?

What are your current rules of thumb to follow for a healthy diet?

How closely do you follow these rules?

What changes have you made in your life since you read *Perfect Body*?

What changes have you experienced in your body?

How do you look and feel?

What effect did *Perfect Body* have on how you look and feel?

What goal did you set for yourself?

What is your time line for achieving your goal?

Has your goal changed? If yes, what is your new goal?

Who can you count on for support?

Have you asked for support? If yes, what kind of support did you ask for? If no, why not?

What kind of support are you getting? Is it valuable?

How do you feel you are doing regarding your goal? Do you feel like you are succeeding? If no, what else can you do to help yourself succeed?

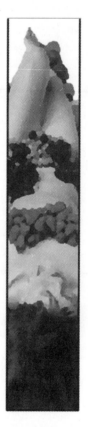

Bibliography

Bibliography

American Cancer Society. Document ID; ACS016. (1995)

American College of Sports Medicine. *Guidelines for Exercise Testing and Prescription.* Philadelphia, PA; Lea & Febiger, 1991

American Medical Association (AMA). "1993 Heart and Stroke Facts." (1994)

Anderson, Bob. *Stretching.* Bolinas, CA; Shelter Books, 1980

Anderson, Walter Truett. *Reality Isn't What It Used To Be.* San Francisco, CA; Harper and Row, 1990.

Arlin, Stephen and Dini, Fouad and Wolfe, David. *Nature's First Law: The Raw Food Diet.* San Diego, CA; Maul Brothers Publishing, 1996

Bach, Richard. *Illusions.* New York, NY; Del Publishing, 1977

Bach, Richard. *Jonathan Livingston Seagull.* New York, NY; Avon Books, 1973

Ballentine, Rudolph. *Diet and Nutrition.* Honesdale, PA; Himalayan International Institute, 1978

Bandler, Richard and Grinder, John. *Frogs into Princes.* Moab, UT; Real People, 1979

Bates, William. *The Bates Method for Better Eyesight Without Glasses.* New York, NY; Henry Holt and Company, 1981

Becker, M. H. *Compliance in Healthcare.* Baltimore, MD; Johns Hopkins University Press, 1979

Berger, B. A. and Felkey, B. G. "A conceptual framework for focusing the teaching of communication skill on compliance gaining strategies." American Journal of Pharmaceutical Education 53 (1989); 259-265

Behavior Training Center. *Hypnotherapy/Behavioral Therapy Training Manual.* Burbank, CA; Behavior Training Center, 1982

Berman, Morris. *The Reenchantment of the World.* Ithaca, NY; Cornell University Press, 1981

Bernard, C. *An Introduction to the Study of Experimental Medicine.* Dover, NY; Paperback, 1957

Bernard, Michael. *Staying Rational in an Irrational World.* New York, NY; Carol Publishing, 1991

Blankenhorn, D. H., Johnson, R. L., Mack, W. J. "The influence of diet on the appearance of new lesions in human coronary arteries." Journal of the American Medical Association 263 (1990); 1646-1652

Bortz II, Walter. *We Live Too Short and Die Too Long.* New York, NY; Banton Books, 1991

Bragg, Patricia. *Nature's Healing System for Better Eyesight.* Santa Barbara, CA; Health Science, 1989

Bragg, Paul C. *The Miracle of Fasting.* Santa Barbara, CA; Health Science, 1983

Bragg, Paul C. *Toxicless Diet Body Purification and Healing System.* Burbank, CA; Health Science, 1967

Bridgman, George B. *The Human Machine.* New York, NY; Dover Publishing Company, 1972

Brown, M. S. and Goldstein, J. L. "A receptor-mediated pathway for cholesterol homeostasis." Science 232 (1986): 34-47

Brunner, D., Weisbort, J., Meshulam, M. "Relation of serum total cholesterol and high-density lipoprotein cholesterol percentage to the incidence of definite coronary events: Twenty year follow-up of the Donolo-Tel Aviv prospective coronary artery disease study." American Journal of Cardiology 59 (1987): 1271-1276

Bruun, Ruth & Bertel. *The Human Body.* New York, NY; Random House, 1982

Burrell, C and Levy, R. *Improving Medication Compliance: Proceedings of a Symposium.* Washington DC (1984): 7-16

Campbell, J. H., Campbell, G. R. Journal of Hypertension. "Cell biology and atherosclerosis" Journal of Hypertension 12 (1994): 129-132

Capra, Fritjof. *The Tao of Physics.* New York, NY

Capra, Fritjof. *The Web of Life.* New York, NY; Anchor Books, 1996

Castelli, W. P. "The epidemiology of coronary heart disease. The Framingham Study" American Journal of Medicine. 76:4-12, 1984

Chen, Phillip. *Inorganic, Organic and Biological Chemistry*. New York, NY; Harper & Row, 1979

Clason, George S. *The Richest Man in Babylon*. New York, NY; Signet Books, 1988

Cousins, Norman. *Anatomy of an Illness*. New York, NY; Bantam Books, 1981

Covey, Stephen. *The 7 Habits of Highly Effective People*. New York, NY; Simon & Schuster, 1990

De Feyter, P. J., Vos, J., Deckers, J. W. "Progression and regression of atherosclerotic plaque." European Heart Journal 16 (1995): 26-30

Duffy, William. *Sugar Blues*. New York, NY; Warner, 1975

Ehret, Arnold. *Mucusless Diet and Healing System*. Yonkers, NY; Ehret Literature Publishing Company, 1989

Eisler, Riane. *The Chalice and the Blade*. San Francisco, CA; Harper, 1988.

Enger, Gibson, Kormelink, Ross, & Smith. *Concepts in Biology*. Dubuque, IO; William C. Brown Company Publishers, 1979

Ennis, R. H. *Critical Thinking*. Upper Saddle River, NJ; Prentice Hall, 1996

Frankl, Viktor E. *Man's Search for Meaning*. New York, NY; Washington Square Press, 1984

Gallo, D. "Educating for Empathy, Reason, and Imagination." Re-Thinking Reason: New Perspectives in Critical Thinking. Albany, NY; State University of New York Press, 1994

Gallo, R. *Body Ecology*. San Francisco, CA; Gallo Publications, 1994

Gawain, Shakti. *Creative Visualization*. New York, NY; Bantam Books, 1982

Gaylord, Chuck and Mitch. *Working Out Without Weights*. New York, NY; William Morrow and Company, Inc., 1985

Gilman, Charlotte Perkins. "The Yellow Wallpaper." The Feminist Press 1973

Golding, Myers, & Sinning. *Y's way to Physical Fitness*. New York, NY; Human Kinetics Publishers, Inc., 1989

Gregory, Dick. *Dick Gregory's Natural Diet for Folks Who Eat*. New York, NY; Harper & Row Publishers, 1973

Hambrecht, R., Niebauer, J., Marburger, C. "Various intensities of leisure time physical activity in patients with coronary artery disease: Effects on cardiorespiratory fitness and progression of atherosclerotic lesions." Journal of American Cardiology 22 (1993): 468-477

Handa, M., Matsusoto, M., Maeda, H., Hougaku, H., Kamada, T. "Ischemic stroke events and carotid atherosclerosis." Stroke 26 (1995): 1781-1786

Hanna, Thomas. *Somatics*. Redding, MA; Addison-Wesley., 1988

Harris, Thomas. *I'm OK, You're OK*. New York, NY; Avon, 1973

Hay, Louise. *You Can Heal Your Life*. Carson, CA; Hay House, 1984.

Haynes, R. B. *Compliance with Therapeutic Regimens*. Baltimore, MD. John Hopkins University Press, 1976

Herrick, J. A. *Critical Thinking: The Analysis of Arguments*. Scottsdale, AZ: Gorsuch Scarisbrick, 1991

Hewitt, James. *The Complete Yoga Book*. New York, NY; Schocken, 1977

Hill, Napoleon. *Think and Grow Rich*. New York, NY; Ballantine Books, 1960

Hoeg J. M. and Kimov, A. N. "In Cholesterol and atherosclerosis: the new is the old rediscovered." American Journal of Cardiology 72 (1993): 1071-1072

Howley , E. & Franks, B. D. *Health/Fitness Instructor's Handbook*. Champaign, IL.: Human Kinetics Pulications, Inc., 1986

Huxley, Aldous. *The Art of Seeing*. Seattle, WA.: Montana Books, 1978

Jensen, Bernard. *Doctor-Patient Handbook*. Escondido, CA.: Bernard Jensen Enterprises, 1984

Jung, Carl. *Memories, Dreams and Reflections*. New York, NY.: Random House, 1989

Kapit, W. & Elson, L. *The Anatomy Coloring Book*. New York, NY.: Harper & Row, 1977

Kapit, Macey & Meisami. *The Physiology Coloring Book*. New York, NY.: Harper Collins, 1987

Keys, A. "Coronary artery disease in seven countries." Circulation 41:42 (1970): 1-211

Keys, Jr. Ken. *Handbook to Higher Consciousness*. Coos Bay, OR.: Love Line Books, 1987

Keys Jr., Ken. *Your Life is a Gift so Make The Most of It*. Coos Bay, OR.: Living Love Publications, 1987

Keys Jr., Ken, and Burkan, Bruce. *How To Make Your Life Work or Why Aren't You Happy?* Coos Bay, OR.: Living Love Publications, 1985

Klein, David. *The Fruits of Healing*. Sebastopol, CA.: Living Nutrition Publications, 1993

Kloss, Jethro. *Back to Eden*. Santa Barbara, CA.: Woodbridge, 1975

Kravette, Stephen. Alternatives to Aging. West Chester, PA.: Whitford Press, 1989

Kusumi, Y., Scanu, A. M., McGill, H. C. "Atherosclerosis in a rhesus monkey with genetic hypercholesterolemia and elevated plasma." Atherosclerosis 99 (1993): 165-174

Lappe, Frances. *Diet for a Small Planet*. New York, NY.: Random House, 1982

Leventhal, H. and Cameron, L. "Behavioral theories and the problem of compliance." Patient Education and Counseling 10 (1987):117-138

Ley, P. "Satisfaction, compliance, and communication." British Journal of Psychology 21 (1982): 241-254

Maffetone, P and Mantel, M. *The High Performance Heart*. Mill Valley, CA: Bicycle Books, 1994

Mander, Jerry. *In the Absence of the Sacred*. San Francisco, CA.: Sierra Club Books, 1991

Mandino, Og. *The Greatest Miracle in the World*. New York, NY.: Bantam Books, 1981

Mandino, Og. *The Greatest Salesman in the World*. New York, NY.: Bantam Books, 1983

McDougall, John. *The McDougall Program*. New York, NY.: Penguin, 1991.

McNaught & Callander. *Illustrated Physiology*. Edinburgh, London.: Churchill Livingstone, 1975

Meichenbaum, D. and Turk, D. C. *Facilitating Treatment Adherence: A Practitioner's Guidebook*. New York, NY: Plenum Press, 1987

Mitchell, Stephen. *Tao to Ching*. New York, NY.: Harper Perennial, 1988

Nieman, David C. *Fitness and Sports Medicine: An Introduction*. Palo Alto, CA.: Bull Publishing Company, 1990

Ornish, D., Brown, S. E., Scherwitz, L. W. "Can lifestyle changes reverse coronary artery disease?" The Lancet 336 (1990): 129-133

Peal, Norman Vincent. *The Power of Positive Thinking*. New York, NY.: Fawcett Crest, 1982

Pearsall, Paul. *Super Joy*. New York, NY.: Doubleday, 1988

Peck, Scott. *The Road Less Traveled*. New York, NY.: Simon & Schuster, 1978

Quackenbush, Thomas R. *Relearning to See*. Berkeley, CA.: North Atlantic Books, 1997

Reinard, J. C. *Introduction to Communication Research*. Madison, WI: Brown and Benchmark, 1994

Remland, M.S., Jones, T.S. "The influence of vocal intensity and touch on compliance gaining." The Journal of Social Psychology 134(1) (1994): 89-97

Robbins, Anthony. *Awaken the Giant Within*. New York, NY: Fireside, 1991

Robbins, Anthony. *Notes from a Friend*. New York, NY: Fireside, 1991

Robbins, Anthony. *Unlimited Power*. New York, NY: Fawcell Columbine Books, 1986

Robbins, John. *Diet for a New America*. Wapole, NH.: Stillpoint Publishing, 1987

Rogers, Carl. *On Becoming a Person*. Boston, MA.: Houghton Mufflin, 1961

Sahtouris, Elisabet. *Gaia The Human Journey from Chaos to Cosmos*. New York, NY.: Pocket Books, 1989

Sapolsky, Robert M. *Why Zebras Don't Get Ulcers*. New York, NY: W. H. Freedom and Company, 1994

Schindler, Lydia. *Understanding the Immune System*. NIH Publication No. 92-529. U.S. Department of Health and Human Services, 1991

Schuler, G., Hambrecht, R., Schlierf, G. "Regular physical exercise and low fat diet: Effects on progression of coronary artery disease." Circulation 86 (1992): 1-11

Shelton, Herbert. *Fasting Can Save Your Life*. Tampa, FL.: American Natural Hygiene Society, 1964

Shelton, Herbert. *Food Combining Made Easy*. San Antonio, TX.: Willow Publishing Company, 1989

Siegel, Bernard. *Love, Medicine, & Miracles*. New York, NY.: Harper & Row, 1986

Silberman, M. *Active Training*. San Diego, CA: Lexington Books, 1990

Silva, Jose. *The Silva Mind Control Method of Mental Dynamics*. New York, NY.: Pocket Books, 1988

Small, B. M. " Progression and regression of atherosclerotic lesions: Insights from lipid physical biochemistry." Arteriosclerosis 8 (1988): 103-129

Stamler J., Wentworth, D., Neaton, J. D. "Is relationship between serum cholesterol and risk of premature death from coronary heart disease continuous or graded?" Journal of the American Medical Association 256 (1986): 2823-2828

Svarstad, B. L. *Growth of Bureaucratic Medicine*. New York, NY: John Wiley and Sons, 1976

Svarstad, B. L. *Application of Social Science to Clinical Medicine and Health Policy*. New Bruswick, NJ.: Rutgers University Press, 1986

Szekely, Edmond. *The Discovery of the Essene Gospel of Peace.* Cartago, Costa Rica.: International Biogenic Society, 1977

Tortora, Gerald, J. *Principles of Human Anatomy.* New York, NY.: Harper Collins Publishers, 1992

Vander, Sherman, Lucino. *Human Physiology.* New York, NY.: McGraw-Hill, 1994

Walker, N. W. *Becoming Younger.* Phoenix, Arizona: Norwalk Press, 1949

Wallston, K. A. and Wallston, B. S. *Social Psychology of Health and Illness.* Hillsdale, NJ. Eribaum Associates, 1982

Warnick, B. and Inch, E. S. *Critical Thinking and Communication.* New York, NY.: Macmillan, 1994

Watts, G. F., Jackson, P., Mandalia, S. "Nutrient intake and progression of coronary artery disease." American Journal of Cardiology 73 (1994): 328-332

Watts, G. F., Mandalia, S., Brunt, J. N. H. "Independent associations between plasma lipoprotein subfraction levels and the course of coronary artery disease in the St. Thomas' Atherosclerosis Regression Study (STARS)." Metabolism 42 (1993): 1461-1467

Weeks, Claire. *Hope and Help for your Nerves.* New York, NY.: Bantam, 1978.

Wittenberg, Henry. *Isometrics Instant Exercise.* New York , NY: Universal Publishing, 1964

Index

Index

J

K

L

M

Sources For A Healthier Lifestyle

Living Nutrition Magazine - a wealth of information on the subject of health and raw food living. For a free introductory copy contact:

David Klein
Living Nutrition
P.O. Box 256
Sebastopol, CA 95473 U.S.A.
(707) 829-8790
e-mail: dklein@living-food.com
http://www.living-foods.com/livingnutrition/

Nature's First Law Catalog - Largest source of books, videos, audio tapes, essays, etc. about raw food living. To receive a free copy contact:

Nature's First Law
P.O. Box 900202
San Diego, CA 92190 U.S.A.
(619) 645-7282
(800) 205-2350 - orders only
e-mail: nature@io-online.com or
Natr1Law@aol.com
Internet Websites:
http://www.io-online.com/~nature